Wound Management

Editors

MICHAEL D. CALDWELL
MICHAEL J. HARL

SURGICAL CLINICS
OF NORTH AMERICA

www.surgical.theclinics.com

Consulting Editor
RONALD F. MARTIN

August 2020 • Volume 100 • Number 4

ELSEVIER

1600 John F. Kennedy Boulevard ● Suite 1800 ● Philadelphia, Pennsylvania, 19103-2899

http://www.surgical.theclinics.com

SURGICAL CLINICS OF NORTH AMERICA Volume 100, Number 4
August 2020 ISSN 0039–6109, ISBN-13: 978-0-323-75494-1

Editor: John Vassallo, j.vassallo@elsevier.com
Developmental Editor: Nicole Congleton

Surgical Clinics of North America (ISSN 0039–6109) is published bimonthly by Elsevier Inc., 360 Park Avenue South, New York, NY 10010-1710. Months of publication are February, April, June, August, October, and December. Business and Editorial Offices: 1600 John F. Kennedy Blvd., Suite 1800, Philadelphia, PA 19103-2899. Periodicals postage paid at New York, NY and additional mailing offices. Subscription prices are $430.00 per year for US individuals, $891.00 per year for US institutions, $100.00 per year for US & Canadian students and residents, $507.00 per year for Canadian individuals, $1130.00 per year for Canadian institutions, $536.00 for international individuals, $1130.00 per year for international institutions and $250.00 per year for foreign students/residents. To receive student/resident rate, orders must be accompanied by name of affiliated institution, date of term, and the *signature* of program/residency coordinator on institution letterhead. Orders will be billed at individual rate until proof of status is received. Foreign air speed delivery is included in all *Clinics* subscription prices. All prices are subject to change without notice. POSTMASTER: Send address changes to *Surgical Clinics*, Elsevier Health Sciences Division, Subscription Customer Service, 3251 Riverport Lane, Maryland Heights, MO 63043. **Customer Service (orders, claims, online, change of address): Telephone: 1-800-654-2452 (U.S. and Canada); 314-447-8871 (outside U.S. and Canada). Fax: 314-447-8029. E-mail: journalscustomerservice-usa@elsevier.com (for print support); journalsonlinesupport-usa@elsevier.com (for online support).**

Reprints. For copies of 100 or more, of articles in this publication, please contact the Commercial Reprints Department, Elsevier Inc., 360 Park Avenue South, New York, New York 10010-1710. Tel. 212-633-3874, Fax: 212-633-3820, E-mail: reprints@elsevier.com.

The Surgical Clinics of North America is also published in Spanish by McGraw-Hill Interamericana Editores S.A., P.O. Box 5-237 06500 Mexico D.F. Mexico; and in Portuguese by Interlivros Edicoes Ltda., Rua Comandante Coelho 1085, CEP 21250, Rio de Janeiro, Brazil; and in Greek by Paschalidis Medical Publications, Athens Greece.

The Surgical Clinics of North America is covered in *MEDLINE/PubMed (Index Medicus), EMBASE/Excerpta Medica, Current Contents/Clinical Medicine, Current Contents/Life Sciences, Science Citation Index,* and *ISI/BIOMED.*

Contributors

CONSULTING EDITOR

RONALD F. MARTIN, MD, FACS
Colonel (Retired), United States Army Reserve, Executive Vice President, Kalispell, Regional Healthcare, Chief Physician Executive, Kalispell Regional Medical Group, Division of HPB Surgery and Surgical Oncology, Kalispell, Montana

EDITORS

MICHAEL D. CALDWELL, MD, PhD FACS
Director, Center for Hyperbaric Medicine and Tissue Repair, Marshfield Clinic, Marshfield, Wisconsin

MICHAEL J. HARL, MD, FACS
Department of Plastic Surgery and Reconstructive Surgery, Marshfield Clinic Health Care System, Marshfield, Wisconsin

AUTHORS

JAMES ABDO, MD
PGY-2, General Surgery, Marshfield Clinic Health System, Marshfield, Wisconsin

JONATHAN F. ARNOLD, MD, ABPM-UHM, CWS-P
Medical Director, Mercy Healing Center, Cedar Rapids, Iowa

ADRIAN BARBUL, MD, FACS
Department of Surgery, Vanderbilt University Medical Center, Department of Surgery, Nashville Veterans Administration Hospital, Nashville, Tennessee

JUSTIN BARR, MD, PhD
Resident, Department of Surgery, Instructor, Department of History, Duke University, Durham, North Carolina

ROBEL T. BEYENE, MD
Department of Surgery, Vanderbilt University Medical Center, Nashville, Tennessee

CHRISTOPHER BIBBO, DO, FACS, FAAOS
Chief, Foot and Ankle Surgery, Limb Salvage, Reconstructive Plastic and Microsurgery, Orthopaedic Trauma, Musculoskeletal Infections, Rubin Institute for Advanced Orthopedics, International Center for Limb Lengthening, Sinai Hospital of Baltimore, Baltimore, Maryland

TIFFANY BROCKE, MD
Johns Hopkins University, Baltimore, Maryland

MICHAEL D. CALDWELL, MD, PhD FACS
Director, Center for Hyperbaric Medicine and Tissue Repair, Marshfield Clinic, Marshfield, Wisconsin

STEPHEN LENTZ DERRYBERRY Jr. MD
Department of Surgery, Vanderbilt University Medical Center, Nashville, Tennessee

ROBERT F. DIEGELMANN, PhD
Distinguished Career Professor of Biochemistry, Virginia Commonwealth University School of Medicine, Richmond, Virginia

STEVEN R. EVELHOCH, MD, DDS, FACS, MMHC, MBA
Chairman, Department of Oral and Maxillofacial Surgery, Marshfield Medical Center, Marshfield, Wisconsin

STEPHANIE R. GOLDBERG, MD
Associate Professor of Surgery, Virginia Commonwealth University School of Medicine, Richmond, Virginia

MICHAEL JAMES HARL, MD, FACS
Department of Plastic Surgery and Reconstructive Surgery, Marshfield Clinic Health Care System, Marshfield, Wisconsin

BRITTANY E. MAYER, DPM
Foot and Ankle Deformity Correction and Orthoplastics Fellow, Rubin Institute for Advanced Orthopedics, International Center for Limb Lengthening, Sinai Hospital of Baltimore, Baltimore, Maryland

LAURA A. MICHETTI, DPM
PGY-3 Resident, Veterans Affairs Maryland Healthcare System, Rubin Institute for Advanced Orthopedics, International Center for Limb Lengthening, Sinai Hospital of Baltimore, Baltimore, Maryland

BRAD T. MORROW, MD
Department of Plastic and Craniomaxillofacial Surgery, Marshfield Clinic Health System, Marshfield, Wisconsin

HOLLY ORTMAN, MD
PGY-2, General Surgery, Marshfield Clinic Health System, Marshfield, Wisconsin

Contents

Chronic wounds present a unique therapeutic challenge to heal. Chronic wounds are colonized with bacteria and the presence of a biofilm that further inhibits the normal wound healing processes, and are locked into a very damaging proinflammatory response. The treatment of chronic wounds requires a coordinated approach, including debridement of devitalized tissue, minimizing bacteria and biofilm, control of inflammation, and the use of specialized dressings to address the specific aspects of the particular nonhealing ulcer.

Wound healing is affected by several factors. Preexisting diagnoses may significantly alter, delay, or inhibit normal wound healing. This is most commonly seen with chronic disorders, such as diabetes and renal failure, but also occurs secondary to aging and substance abuse. Less commonly, genetic or inflammatory disorders are the cause of delayed wound healing. In some cases, it is not the illness, but the treatment that can inhibit wound healing. This is seen in patients getting chemotherapy, radiation, steroids, methotrexate, and a host of other medications. Understanding these processes may help treat or avoid wound healing problems.

Chronic wounds often are the result of bone deformities, compounded by musculotendinous and ligamentous imbalance. Sensory neuropathy places patients at greater risk for acute wounds to develop into chronic wounds. Etiologies of these deforming forces include Charcot neuroarthropathy, trauma, and congenital and acquired neuromuscular disorders. Management of these deformities ranges from simple relief of pressure with soft inserts to bracing for mechanical instability. Correction of more complex deformities requires resection of bone, osteotomies, fusions, and external fixation. Tendon and ligament imbalance must be addressed at all levels of deformity. Postoperatively, patients must be re-evaluated for continuation of orthoses and bracing.

In this review, the author summarizes the role of biofilm formation in chronic nonhealing wound infections along with characteristics of biofilm formation, diagnosis, detection, and treatment. Because biofilms are still not clearly understood, treatment and diagnosis are currently difficult.

This article reviews techniques for wound coverage that are not amenable to simple linear closure. The relevant anatomy and classification of flaps is discussed, as well as specific techniques for successful flap design.

Cellular and/or tissue-based products (CTPs) have advanced greatly in the past several decades and improve the ability to heal wounds more efficiently. Products can be characterized as nonviable cells, tissue based, animal; nonviable cells, tissue based, human; viable human cells, cultured in vitro, animal substrate; viable human cells, cultured in vitro, synthetic substrate; viable human cells, noncultured, intact tissue. There are approximately 77 different CTPs at the time of this writing, with many more being investigated. Cellular and/or tissue-based product selection, application, postapplication course, and patient selection depend on patient attributes, CTP specifications, and surgeon preference.

This review of the literature concerning bacteria, antibiotics and tissue repair shows there are extensive data supporting microbial interference with wound healing once bacterial burden exceeds 104 CFU per unit of measure, The mechanism of bacterial interference lies largely in prolonging the inflammatory phase of tissue repair. Reducing the microbial bioburden allows tissue repair to continue. Systemic and topical antimicrobials appear critical to reducing the bioburden and facilitating repair. The current controversy over the use of antimicrobials in patients with chronically infected wounds, in particular, revolves around the definition of infection. The reliance on classic clinical signs of inflammation to support antimicrobial use in these patients is tenuous due to the lack of correlation of these signs with the microbial burden known to impair tissue repair.

The discipline of reconstructive surgery has been slow to accept the role of hyperbaric oxygen therapy (HBOT) as an adjunct to surgery, despite clinical and experimental data showing potential benefits. Obstacles prevent this acceptance; one of the most potent is surgeon bias. This article attempts to lessen this bias by reviewing the benefits of HBOT in conditions where there is uniform acceptance of its role, such as carbon monoxide poisoning and decompression illness. It demonstrates that these conditions have similar pathophysiologic derangements to conditions commonly encountered by the reconstructive/wound care surgeon, including crush injuries, compartment syndrome, compromised flaps, and thermal burns.

Since the dawn of humanity, wounds have afflicted humans, and healers have held responsibility for treating them. This article tracks the evolution of wound care from antiquity to the present, highlighting the roles of surgeons, scientists, culture, and society in the ever-changing management of traumatic and iatrogenic injuries.

Peripheral arterial disease (PAD) affects many individuals worldwide and is associated with increased morbidity and mortality. Controversy exists on whether or not to screen asymptomatic patients. Further complicating this is that many patients with a chronic lower extremity wound are often asymptomatic. PAD and traditional noninvasive vascular studies may be inaccurate in providing a correct diagnosis. A review of current and novel vascular assessment modalities along with their benefits and limitations are presented here. A combination of these vascular assessments may help improve accuracy in diagnosis, providing timely care to those patients in need.

SURGICAL CLINICS
OF NORTH AMERICA

SERIES OF RELATED INTEREST

Advances in Surgery
https://www.advancessurgery.com/
Surgical Oncology Clinics
https://www.surgonc.theclinics.com/
Thoracic Surgery Clinics
http://www.thoracic.theclinics.com/

THE CLINICS ARE AVAILABLE ONLINE!
Access your subscription at:
www.theclinics.com

Foreword
Wound Healing

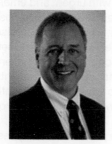

Ronald F. Martin, MD, FACS
Consulting Editor

There is an adage that time heals all wounds: would that it were so. I suppose if some-one were to take an extremist view, one might consider that saying is true in the way one might believe that "all bleeding stops." I think it can be readily said that time, in and of itself, is not the most significant contributor to wound healing and may actually be working against some people. The process of wound healing is complex, involving many interrelated biological processes, host factors, and environmental contributions. Furthermore, there are the wounds that will heal well given time and those wounds that will never heal unless they are actively managed to do so, which, ironically sometimes means getting the wound closed quickly.

I don't know how society will be functioning by the time this issue of the *Surgical Clinics* is distributed. At the time of my writing this, the United States is largely under varying degrees of sheltering-in-place orders and social-distancing rules to attempt to manage the COVID-19 pandemic. A few states are beginning to modify their posi-tions. We don't know how that will change things at this moment. Where I am in Montana, we have been particularly fortunate in that the very nature of the state pro-vides for "social distancing" as a norm. Also, we were able to see the challenges hitting Seattle and New York City long before we had significant disease burden and were able to adopt robust measures in a timely fashion. Some of these measures were sig-nificant restrictions of appointment and procedure availability for our patients.

Health care systems around the world had to alter their approaches to the practice of medicine. For us, we had to make many changes, but perhaps one of the most lasting ones will be our marked increase in the use of telehealth measures. One of my admin-istrative colleagues, Jason Spring, first suggested to our group that he believed one of the most important things the COVID-19 pandemic will be remembered for was the conversion of American medicine to greater use of telehealth. I think he will be right. Our use was well under 4% of visits prior to the pandemic, and by the time of this writing, we have some clinics at 40% telehealth visits, with expectations to climb. Of course, this phenomenon was driven by many factors, not the least of which was a change in the rules for billing for services.

Virtual life has become a "real thing" for many of us. Telehealth, virtual conferences, remote workstations, and so forth have all become commonplace. Still, sometimes there is no virtual replacement for the real thing. We as surgeons are more acutely aware of that than almost anyone. Certainly, acute care surgery with urgent and emergent operations went on as best it could with modified processes and protective postures. Scheduled procedures (frequently described by that horribly imprecise descriptor "elective") were deferred if possible based on some assessment of their acuity and the safety of waiting. In the middle of those concepts lies the patient who is not in peril of life but cannot suspend their course of treatment. Some patients with cancer fit into this category, but also patients with chronic wounds often fit into this category. These patients did not always have a clear-cut "position" within the proposed hierarchies of needs assessment.

As travel became more restrictive for patients and health care providers of all types, numerous workarounds were created to try to fill in shortfalls in care. Some of them were ingenious and a real testament to the creativity of a people in distress. For many patients who had chronic nonhealing wounds, we tried to combine either self-wound care or assisted-wound care in the home environment with digital support to relay images for assessment by knowledgeable persons. In some instances, this was very helpful, but it was not a replacement for seeing and examining patients in person and for using the other adjunctive tools that we normally have in hospital environments.

As stated at the outset, wound healing is complicated. In some regards, the least important piece of the puzzle is the wound. It is surprising to many that the bigger pieces of the puzzle are the systemic issues. When I would care for people with chronic wounds at our wound center, it never ceased to amaze me how few patients with a wound that had been nonhealing for months (or longer) had not had even the most rudimentary evaluation of perfusion to an area. Or other patients with chronic disease that was poorly controlled had not had measures taken to improve their glucose control or oxygenation.

This issue of the *Surgical Clinics*, edited by Drs Michael Caldwell and Michael Harl, gives the reader a detailed and comprehensive review of how all the clinical, technical, and environmental factors can be fit together to maximize the chance of getting chronic wounds closed and healed. I am particularly grateful that they were able to consolidate the production of this issue during the period of maximum life disturbance from the pandemic.

As in life in general, many things are more complex than they appear to be on the surface. Wound healing is an excellent example of that. It is affected at the most molecular level as biological processes and affected at the most altitudinal level as a problem of socioeconomic dislocation for many. Nonhealing wounds hobble our patients literally and hobble our society with other substantial costs. If we are to improve life and quality of life for these patients, we need to address as many of these issues at all levels as best we can. This collection of reviews should help one do that or at least advocate for it.

We at the *Surgical Clinics* wish everyone good health and safety. I hope that by the time you read this, your own personal situation will be markedly improved and you will be able to enjoy your health and society with loved ones. Thank you all for your support of this series. We are grateful for you.

Ronald F. Martin, MD, FACS
Colonel (retired)
United States Army Reserve
Kalispell Regional Healthcare
Kalispell Regional Medical Group
Division of HPB Surgery and Surgical Oncology
310 Sunnyview Lane
Kalispell, MT 59901, USA

E-mail address:
rfmcescna@gmail.com

Preface

Wound Healing: A Call for Engagement

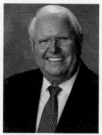   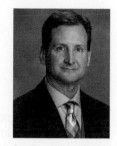

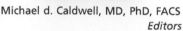

Michael d. Caldwell, MD, PhD, FACS   Michael J. Harl, MD, FACS
Editors

This issue of *Surgical Clinics* is designed to give the reader a summary of important aspects of tissue repair. The authors have prepared excellent articles that amply address difficult issues in origin and persistence of chronic wounds, and an update on modern methods to heal them. We appreciate the opportunity to host this issue given by Dr Ron Martin, the forbearing Consulting Editor of *Surgical Clinics*. We also greatly appreciate the contributions of each of the article authors and hope that the reader will find their efforts to be as outstanding as we believe them to be. We hope that this issue will provide the reader with new and intriguing knowledge of wounds and wound healing and surgeons with an impetus to overcome the temptation of minimal intervention and actively engage in reducing the morbidity of chronic wounds.

Ten years ago in the issue on Wounds and Wound Management for *Surgical Clinics*, the first article was entitled "Wound Surgery." The casual reader may not have made much of this title, but for surgeons involved in wound care, we believe it means everything. This is because it stands in stark contrast to the philosophy of much of current tissue repair practice, which focuses on "wound care."

We have adopted a motto for our practice: "We don't care for wounds—we close them." This statement underscores the philosophical difference between wound surgeons and other providers involved in wound care. This sentiment is further contained in OP Hampton's statement, "Every open wound needs and deserves surgery. Either it is ready for closure by suture or skin graft or it needs debridement to prevent or eliminate sepsis and the destruction of living tissue and to prepare it for closure." Yet, due to a combination of surgeon indifference and ubiquitous outpatient "wound clinics," surgeon involvement with wound care has declined. The void has been filled with well-meaning providers who frequently lack surgical support and therefore must rely on available dressings and bioengineered "produits du jour" to achieve tissue repair by secondary intention.

Surg Clin N Am 100 (2020) xiii–xiv
https://doi.org/10.1016/j.suc.2020.06.001
0039-6109/20/© 2020 Published by Elsevier Inc.

The loss of surgeons further hampers the world of wound care due to the surgeon's ability to debride necrotic tissue and pseudo-science alike.

The above-mentioned article ended with "a call for closure." This preface will conclude with a request that is far more basic, and that is, a call for engagement. In our opinion, both the specialty of surgery and patients with chronic wounds will pay a heavy price if surgeons continue to withdraw from the arena of wound care.

Michael D. Caldwell, MD, PhD, FACS
Marshfield Clinic Center for
Hyperbaric Medicine and Tissue Repair

Michael J. Harl, MD, FACS
Marshfield Clinic Department of
Plastic and Reconstructive Surgery

E-mail addresses:
caldwell.michael@marshfieldclinic.org (M.D. Caldwell)
Harl.michael@marshfieldclinic.org (M.J. Harl)

What Makes Wounds Chronic

Stephanie R. Goldberg, MD[a], Robert F. Diegelmann, PhD[b],*

KEYWORDS

- Chronic wound • Ulcer • Biofilm • Bacteria • Inflammation • Proteases • Cytokines
- Wound healing

KEY POINTS

- Ischemia is a common denominator in chronic ulcers. The result of ischemia is tissue injury, necrosis, and the development of open wounds that are quickly colonized by bacteria.
- The infection sets the stage for chronic and uncontrolled inflammation. As the host's inflammatory cells try to remove the damaged tissue, reactive oxygen species and proteases are released, causing further tissue damage.
- The proinflammatory response is perpetuated by the formation of a biofilm that walls off and protects the bacteria and the inflamed ulcer site.
- Because of the raging inflammatory environment, residual connective tissue cells have decreased mitogenic activity and become senescent.
- This vicious cycle of inflammation and tissue destruction persists until aggressive clinical strategies are used to remove bacteria, damaged and necrotic tissue and reduce inflammation.

INTRODUCTION

The wound healing process consists of a carefully coordinated sequence of events after a cutaneous injury leading to regeneration of the skin protective barrier.[1] After an initial insult, wounds that fail to progress through the stages of wound healing within a 3-month period of time are deemed chronic wounds.[2] Chronic wounds are characterized by a prolonged and sustained inflammatory phase that prevents dermal and epidermal cells from responding to chemical signals.[3] Most chronic wounds begin with small tissue insults, including minor trauma or skin tears and insect bites. In the setting of comorbidities including diabetes and arterial insufficiency that inhibit blood flow, these wound often evolve into chronic nonhealing wounds. With the increasing elderly population combined with increased worldwide risk of diabetes, chronic wounds represent a significant contributor to health care costs and morbidity.

a Virginia Commonwealth University School of Medicine, PO Box 980454, 1200 East Broad Street, Richmond, VA 23219, USA; b Virginia Commonwealth University School of Medicine, PO Box 980614, 1100 East Marshall Street, Richmond, VA 23298-0614, USA
* Corresponding author.
E-mail address: robert.diegelmann@vcuhealth.org

Surg Clin N Am 100 (2020) 681–693
https://doi.org/10.1016/j.suc.2020.05.001
0039-6109/20/© 2020 Elsevier Inc. All rights reserved.

TYPES OF CHRONIC WOUNDS

Chronic wounds are classified into vascular ulcers (venous and arterial), diabetic ulcers, and pressure ulcers, all of which have different causes but can lead to nonhealing wounds. Most chronic wounds fail to progress beyond the inflammatory phase of wound healing and are often impacted by the presence of infection[4] drug-resistant biofilms (see Steven R. Evelhoch's article, "Biofilm and Chronic Non-Healing Wound Infections," in this issue),[5] and a loss of response to chemotactic stimuli[6] that preclude them from healing. Although there are similarities among these nonhealing wounds, they differ in terms of the mechanism underlying their inability to heal.[7]

Vascular Ulcers

Vascular ulcers can arise from either venous or arterial insufficiency. Venous ulcers are preceded by symptoms of heaviness and pain in the legs and often associated with swelling, varicose veins, and areas of hyperpigmentation owing to hemosiderin, a breakdown product of hemoglobin. Lipodermatosclerosis, an inflammation of the layer of fat under the epidermis of the limb, occurs when skin and subcutaneous tissue are replaced by fibrinous scar before ulcer formation. Venous ulcers then occur when incompetent valves or obstruction in the superficial and deep veins result in a backflow of blood, leading to increased venous pressure, changes in blood vessel permeability with fibrin, plasma, and red blood cell leakage into the interstitial space. These entities serve as chemoattractants for leukocytes infiltration into the area.[3] Fibrin accumulation downregulates collagen synthesis and accumulates in the form of pericapillary fibrin cuffs.[8] There are 3 main theories regarding the development of ulcers in venous insufficiency.[9] The fibrin cuff theory supports the trapping of various factors that stimulate prolonged inflammation and interfere with oxygen tissue diffusion, further impacting the normal wound healing cascade. The leukocyte entrapment theory suggests that venous hypertension leads to a decrease in the pressure gradient in the capillaries such that blood moves sluggishly and increases the adherence of blood cells to the endothelium resulting in the release of inflammatory mediators such as tumor necrosis factor α (TNFα) that upregulates the adhesion molecules, intercellular adhesion molecule-1, vascular cell adhesion molecule-1, and reactive oxygen species causing ischemia and ulceration.[10] Last, the microangiopathy theory suggests there is occlusion of capillaries by microthrombi leading to poor oxygenation. These associated venous skin changes predispose patients to developing venous stasis ulcers in the setting of minor trauma.

Arterial ulcers result from arterial insufficiency from atherosclerosis that prevents adequate blood flow perfusion leading to tissue ischemia and necrosis.[11,12] These ulcers may be associated with advanced age, smoking, diabetes mellitus, hypertension, dyslipidemia, family history, obesity, and a sedentary lifestyle. There are multiple theories regarding the pathogenesis of ischemic leg ulcers, but all coalesce into decreased tissue oxygenation secondary to poor blood flow.

Pressure Ulcers

Pressure ulcers occur from tissue ischemia from sustained direct pressure and shearing forces applied to skin. These ulcers are most common in patients with poor mobility and neuropathies, although they can be worsened by a patient with concomitant venous or arterial insufficiency.

Although friction and shear stress cause direct epidermal and dermal skin changes and subepidermal breaks in skin, the mechanical load causes changes in interstitial fluid content, ultimately leading to tissue necrosis. There is a significant upregulation of inflammatory markers in the adipose tissue in response to reperfusion injury related hypoxia and reoxygenation, suggesting that the adipocytes may drive this inflammatory response. Pressure ulcers are characterized by an excessive density of neutrophils.[13]

Diabetic Ulcers

Diabetic ulcers occur in the setting of peripheral neuropathy in which patients are unable to recognize repeated minor trauma to the legs. The mechanism underlying the pathogenesis of diabetic ulcers includes elevated glucose levels causing increased levels of reactive oxygen species, nitric oxide blockade, DNA alternation, elevation protein kinase C, ischemia, and inflammation.[14] Peripheral arterial disease further contributes to disease pathogenesis owing to decreased capillary size, thickening of the basement membrane, and arteriolar hyalinosis.[15] Persistent hyperglycemia also causes endothelial dysfunction and smooth muscle abnormalities, with resulting vasoconstriction[16] The chronicity and poor wound healing associated with diabetic ulcers is multifactorial and includes abnormalities in growth factor production, angiogenesis, cell migration and proliferation, collagen deposition, and extracellular matrix remodeling by proteases.[17–19]

NORMAL WOUND HEALING

The process of normal wound healing consists of 4 key phases in which cells and an extracellular matrix provide a framework for collagen growth and deposition.[1] The 4 phases of wound healing include hemostasis, inflammation, proliferation, and remodeling (**Fig. 1**) and relies on chemical mediators including growth factors, chemokines, and inhibitors. In the hemostasis phase, the process begins with vasoconstriction followed by platelet activation by collagen binding to an extracellular matrix. The platelets release chemical factors, including fibronectin, thrombospondin, sphingosine-1-

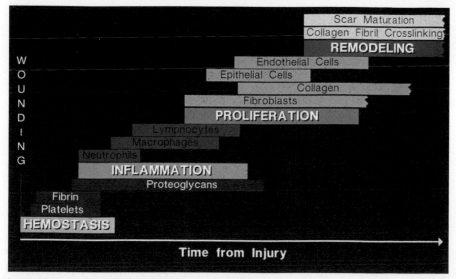

Fig. 1. Phases of normal wound healing. Cellular and molecular events during normal wound healing progress through 4 major, integrated, phases: hemostasis, inflammation, proliferation, and remodeling. (*From* Cohen IK, Diegelmann RF, Linblad WJ. Wound Healing: Biochemical & Clinical Aspects. Philadelphia, PA: W.B. Saunders Co.; 1992; with permission.)

phosphate, and von Willebrand's factor, which aid in ongoing control of bleeding in the wound.[20–22] Insoluble fibrin forms a provisional matrix to which platelets adhere and form a plug or clotlike structure[23] (**Fig. 2**).

Wounds then progress within 24 hours after injury to the next phase of wound healing called the inflammatory phase lasting until postinjury day 4. This phase is characterized by cell-mediated removal of bacteria and devitalized tissue through the migration of neutrophils and macrophages to allow for subsequent collagen deposition by fibroblasts and neovascularization[24] (**Fig. 3**). Neutrophils bind to specialized cell adhesion molecules on endothelial cells to then marginate and squeeze through leaky cell junctions into the interstitial space through a process of pavementing and diapedesis. Neutrophil migration is termed chemotaxis and is mediated by both chemokines and bacterial presence within a wound. Neutrophils generate reactive oxygen species via the enzyme myeloperoxidase, phagocytize foreign debris, and release matrix metalloproteinases (MMPs), which further digest surrounding necrotic tissue. Activated macrophages also function as phagocytic cells and release proteases to further digest injured tissues.

The transition to the next phase of wound healing occurs when neutrophils release IL-1 and TNFα to activate fibroblasts and epithelial cells and macrophages release multiple growth factors including platelet-derived growth factor, transforming growth factor-β, TNFα, fibroblast growth factor, insulin-like growth factor-1, and IL-6. The critical phase of wound healing, called the proliferative phase, occurs between postinjury days 4 and 21 and heavily relies on fibroblast proliferation and migration. This phase is characterized by collagen synthesis, deposition and cross-linking, and formation of a reconstituted extracellular matrix by the addition of proteoglycans (**Fig. 4**). Open wounds begin to contract through specialized cells called myofibroblasts.[25] The presence of MMPs from inflammatory cells and fibroblasts allows for ongoing collagen remodeling but they are regulated by specific inhibitors, called tissue inhibitors of MMPs. The net result is that there is more collagen deposition than destruction.[26,27]

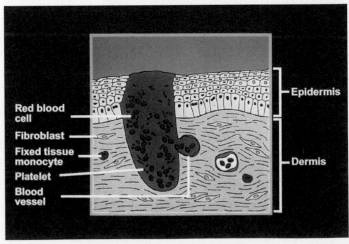

Fig. 2. Hemostasis phase. At the time of injury, the fibrin clot forms the provisional wound matrix and platelets release multiple growth factors that initiate the repair process. (*From* Chandawarkar R, Miller MJ. Wound Healing. In: Mulholland MW, Lillemoe KD, Doherty GM et al. Greenfield's Surgery: Scientific Principles & Practice. 6th ed. Philadelphia, PA: J. B. Lippincott & Co.; 1993; with permission.)

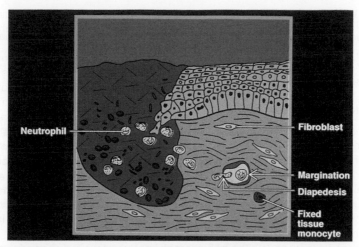

Fig. 3. Inflammatory phase. Within 1 day after an injury, the inflammatory phase is initiated by neutrophils that attach to endothelial cells in the vessel walls surrounding the wound (margination), change shape and move through the cell junctions (diapedesis), and migrate to the wound site (chemotaxis). (*From* Chandawarkar R, Miller MJ. Wound Healing. In: Mulholland MW, Lillemoe KD, Doherty GM et al. Greenfield's Surgery: Scientific Principles & Practice. 6th ed. Philadelphia, PA: J. B. Lippincott & Co.; 1993; with permission.)

The last phase of wound healing is called the remodoling phase, goes on for years, and occurs once all extracellular matrix components have been deposited in the wound site (**Fig. 5**). The final wound appears as a scar with approximately 80% of the original tensile strength of normal tissue. In this phase, the initial type III collagen that was deposited, is replaced by type 1 collagen and cross-linked.[28]

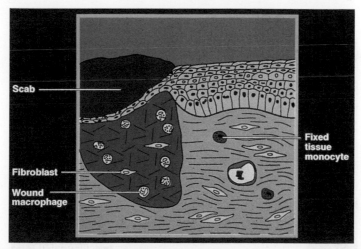

Fig. 4. Proliferation phase. Fixed tissue monocytes activate, move into the site of injury, transform into activated wound macrophages that kill bacteria, release proteases that remove denatured extracellular matrix, and secrete growth factors that stimulate fibroblast, epidermal cells, and endothelial cells to proliferate and produce scar tissue. (*From* Chandawarkar R, Miller MJ. Wound Healing. In: Mulholland MW, Lillemoe KD, Doherty GM et al. Greenfield's Surgery: Scientific Principles & Practice. 6th ed. Philadelphia, PA: J. B. Lippincott & Co.; 1993; with permission.)

CHRONIC WOUND HEALING

Chronic wounds fail to progress through the organized phases of wound healing in a timely manner.[2] Although they differ in etiology, chronic wounds are typically characterized by excessive levels of proinflammatory cytokines, proteases, reactive oxygen species, senescent cells, bioburen, and a deficiency of functional stem cells.[29]

Inflammation: Bacteria and Biofilms in Chronic Wounds

Bacteria have the ability to both colonize and infect wounds, causing major problems in the chronic wound setting. Most chronic wounds are polymicrobial in nature with a preponderance of *Staphylococcus* and *Pseudomonas* species.[30] Anaerobic bacteria are found in a relative abundance in chronic wounds, which are continually exposed to high levels of oxygen.[31] Interestingly, there is a paucity of *Corynebacterium*, a commensal bacteria, in these wounds. Commensal bacteria have long been shown to benefit the host organism by educating the host adaptive response and inhibiting the growth of pathogenic bacteria[32,33] (recent data have shown coryneform bacteria to be pathogenic in wounds). The polymicrobial nature of wound allows for microbial diversity and heterogeneity with in a wound, further challenging the wound's ability to heal.

To strengthen their antimicrobial resistance, planktonic bacteria evolved to create biofilms. Biofilms are formed when bacterial cells attach to a surface and use quorum-sensing molecules to induce changes in gene expression, which ultimately creates a barrier consisting of predominately exopolymers, with some residual bacterial cells. The biofilm consists of 85% exopolymers, including polysaccharides, proteins, and nucleic acids, combined with 15% bacteria and form the mature biofilm. Biofilms are consistently polymicrobial with planktonic cells leaving the area to find additional areas to colonize. Steven R. Evelhoch's article, "Biofilm and Chronic Non-Healing Wound Infections," in this issue focuses on role of biofilms in wound healing.

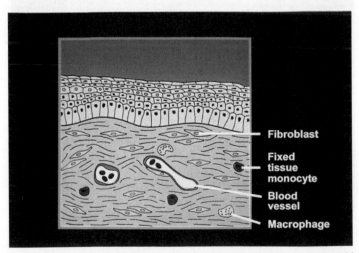

Fig. 5. Remodeling phase. The initial, disorganized scar tissue is slowly replaced by a matrix that more closely resembles the organized extracellular matrix of normal skin. (*From* Chandawarkar R, Miller MJ. Wound Healing. In: Mulholland MW, Lillemoe KD, Doherty GM et al. Greenfield's Surgery: Scientific Principles & Practice. 6th ed. Philadelphia, PA: J. B. Lippincott & Co.; 1993; with permission.)

Biofilms stimulate the host immune response

Biofilms have been shown to be even more recalcitrant than bacteria to the host immune response, making them an even greater challenge for chronic wounds than bacteria alone. Leukocytes within the wound have difficulty penetrating and maneuvering through the biofilm and have an impaired ability to produce reactive oxygen species.[34] This property also prevents phagocytosis of bacteria through normal wound healing pathways. The structural exopolymer of the biofilm has been suggested to evade aspects of the host inflammatory response by further blocking complement activation, suppressing the lymphoproliferative response, and impairing the ability of opsonins on bacterial walls to be detected by phagocytes. There seems to be heterogeneity in biofilms, likely depending on the specific pathogenic micro-organisms.

Biofilms directly resist antimicrobial therapy

By creating and incorporating into biofilms, bacterial cells create an environment where they have decreased metabolic activity, thus rendering themselves less effective against antimicrobial agents that target metabolically active cells.[35] An additional mechanism of resistance is that the exopolysaccharide in the biofilm functions as a mechanical barrier to protect bacteria from antimicrobials and the host immune cells.[36] Biofilms allow for the transfer of plasmid-mediated antimicrobial resistance genes among bacteria within a biofilm that not only adds to the heterogeneity of the wound, but also provides added resistance. Some biofilms are thought to have concentration gradients to minimize the impact of antibiotics and antiseptics, whereas some biofilms may be eradicated after antimicrobial therapy only to have persister cells stimulate regrowth of biofilm once these agents have been removed. Biofilms may possess an additional evolutionary response to antimicrobial therapy by developing thicker mucoid-like phenotypes in response to some antimicrobial therapies.

Biofilms stimulate chronic inflammation

Biofilms are present in nearly 60% of chronic wound but only 10% of acute wounds, and notably stimulate chronic inflammation in the chronic setting. Stimulation of the immune system when unable to effectively eradicate infection can lead to worsening of chronic inflammation and perpetuate the cycle of the chronic wound. This phenomenon occurs through gene expression, which induces inflammation to promote plasma leakage from local capillaries for nutrition.[37] Additionally, biofilms contribute to wound bed senescence cause by oxidative stress and protease-mediated degradation of receptors and cytokines. This leads to alterations in host cell cytoskeleton, inhibition of mitosis, and apoptosis.

PROTEASES

Wounds produce MMPs, calcium-dependent zinc-containing enzymes, that, together with their inhibitors, play key role in the regulation of extracellular matrix deposition and degradation.[38] MMPs can be divided into 7 groups based on the substrate preference and domain organization: (1) collagenases, (2) gelatinases, (3) stromelysins, (4) matrilysins, (5) metalloelastases, (6) membrane-type MMPs, and (7) other MMPs.

Overexpression of MMPs causes damage to the extracellular matrix and drives the underlying pathology of chronic, nonhealing wounds. Overproduction of MMPs also destroys vital growth factors such as platelet-derived growth factor and transforming growth factor-β necessary for wound healing. This overproduction results in an unregulated, continuous inflammatory phase for chronic nonhealing wounds. In normal tissue, there are very low levels of MMPs. In injured tissue, fibroblasts, keratinocytes, endothelial, and inflammatory cells secrete MMPs in response to cytokines, hormones, and other cell types in the extracellular matrix. Cytokines and growth factors known to transcriptionally activate MMPs include transforming growth factor-β, vascular endothelial growth factor, epidermal growth factor, interleukins and interferons, all of which are important in wound healing.[39] Overexpression of MMP-1 delays re-epithelization and is known to be elevated in chronic wounds associated with diabetic foot ulcers.[19,40]

Neutrophil-derived MMP-8 has been associated with chronic wounds.[41] Circulating neutrophils respond to a site of injury and secrete proinflammatory mediators to recruit other inflammatory cells. Neutrophils subsequently undergo apoptosis with phagocytosis by macrophages, which ends the inflammatory phase of wound healing in normal wounds. However, in chronic wounds, neutrophils continue to recruit additional inflammatory cells to the wound bed, leading to ongoing inflammation. Extracellular release of reactive oxygen species and proteases also cause ongoing tissue damage, which further impairs wound healing through defective collagen deposition, decreased wound strength, and delayed re-epithelialization. Protease function is also regulated by multiple protease inhibitors stored in neutrophils. α1-Antitrypsin has been shown to be degraded in chronic wounds, which is thought to contribute to excess serine protease activity in chronic wounds. Fibronectin degradation in chronic wounds depends on the relative levels of elastase, α-1-proteinase inhibitor, and α-2-macroglobulin.[42,43]

PROINFLAMMATORY MEDIATORS (IL-8, IL-6, AND TUMOR NECROSIS FACTOR-α)

Although there are a number of proinflammatory mediators and factors responsible for the chronicity and prolonged inflammation in chronic ulcers, there are several that are major players.[7] IL-8 is a well-known chemoattractant and activator of neutrophils and has a prominent role in chronic ulcers.[44] One of the hallmarks of inflammation is the excessive presence of neutrophils that release several damaging proteases such as MMP 8 and elastase.[13] IL-6 is an interesting and a multifunctional cytokine that elicits a spectrum of responses.[45] It is a potent proinflammatory signal and contributes to the chronicity of chronic ulcers.[46,47] TNFα is another well-known proinflammatory cytokine that has been shown to cause tissue damage in sites of infection.[48] As with IL-6 and IL-8, TNFα also has a critical role in the chronicity of nonhealing ulcers.[49]

TREATMENT OF CHRONIC WOUNDS: HOW TO BREAK THE INFLAMMATORY CYCLE
Debridement, Infection/Inflammation, Moisture Management, Edge/Environment, Support Products and Services: A Holistic Approach to the Management of Chronic Wounds

The debridement, infection/inflammation, moisture management, edge/environment, support products and services wound care guideline was developed as an overall approach to managing patient's wounds and addressing underlying comorbidities.[50] The infection/inflammation, moisture management, edge/environment, support products and services process consists of a comprehensive approach to wound bed preparation, control of infection and inflammation, and maintaining an appropriate moisture balance within the wound (**Fig. 6**).

Specifically, wounds are assessed for the presence of devitalized, infected, and/or inflamed tissue that may inhibit the wound healing process. Ongoing within the chronic wounds are then addressed by physical examination for heat, pain, redness, and swelling. Pain is a reliable marker of infection. Debridement of this devitalized tissue removes areas with high bacterial loads, biofilm, and helps to reinvigorate the wound healing process in tissue with a higher oxygen tension.

Removal of this tissue also removes the bacteria, proteases, inflammatory mediators, and hyperproliferative wound edges that stall a wound in a prolonged

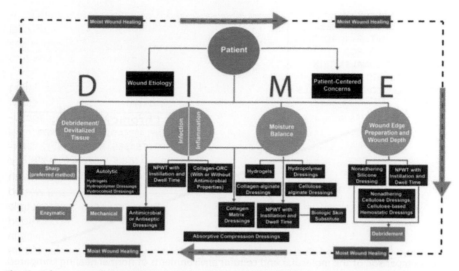

Fig. 6. Schematic of devitalized tissue, infection/inflammation, moisture balance, and edge preparation wound treatment strategy. NPWT, negative pressure wound therapy; ORC, oxidized regenerated cellulose. (*From* Snyder RJ, Fife C, Moore Z. Components and Quality Measures of DIME (Devitalized Tissue, Infection/Inflammation, Moisture Balance, and Edge Preparation) in Wound Care. *Adv Skin Wound Care*. 2016;29(5):205-215; with permission.)

inflammatory phase. Removal of chronic hyper granulation tissue is necessary; it has been shown to decrease the amount of antibiotics that can reach a wound infection and prolong the wound healing process. Wound debridement can be in the form of sharp debridement, mechanical debridement with negative pressure wound therapy with instillation and dwell time, or autolytic debridement through hydrogels and hydrocolloid dressings, depending on the extent of devitalized tissue burden. The presence of inflammation is addressed by looking for underlying causes including malignancy, vasculitis, vasculopathy, and pathergy in the form of pyoderma gangrenosum and biopsy when necessary. Collagen matrix dressings may be used to facilitate a decrease in wound inflammation. Maintaining wound moisture balance is also an important aspect of chronic wound healing. The wound bed is assessed through an evaluation of the quality, odor, and consistency of drainage both within the wound and the surrounding periwound tissue. A moist environment is necessary to promote growth factors, cytokines, and chemokine function in a wound. Too much moisture, however, can lead to periwound maceration and stall the wound care process within the wound bed. A dry wound bed, resulting from exposure of the wound to air, leads to desiccation and necrosis and perpetuates the cycle of poor wound healing.

ADJUNCTIVE THERAPIES

Many adjunctive wound care therapies have been developed to facilitate the healing of chronic wounds. Topical antibiotics may be used to minimize bacterial infection with bacterial threshold of 10^5. Silver- and iodine-impregnated dressings may also be used to control bacterial load on an ongoing basis. Moist occlusive dressings help to create an environment with low oxygen tension and facilitate re-epithelization through activation of hypoxia-inducible factor 1.[51]

Negative pressure wound therapy has been widely used to facilitate chronic wound healing by 4 primary mechanisms (macrodeformation, microdeformation, fluid

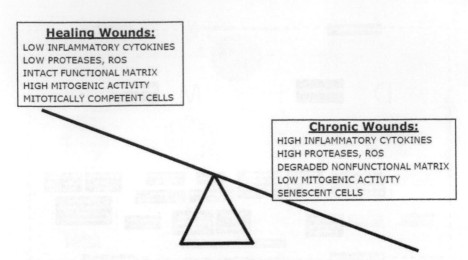

Fig. 7. Comparison of the molecular and cellular environments of normal healing compared with chronic wounds. Elevated levels of cytokines and proteases in chronic wounds reduce mitogenic activities and response of wound cells thus impairing healing. ROS, reactive oxygen species. (*From* Schultz GS, Chin GA, Moldawer L, et al. Principles of Wound Healing. In: Fitridge R, Thompson M, eds. Mechanims of Vascular Disease: A Reference Book for Vascular Specialists [Internet]. Adelaide, Australia: University of Adelaide Press; 2011; with permission.)

removal, and alteration of the wound environment) and various secondary mechanisms (including neurogenesis, angiogenesis, modulation of inflammation, and alterations in bioburden).[52,53]

SUMMARY

Fig. 7 summarizes this article by showing the comparison of the molecular and cellular environments of normal healing compared with chronic wounds. Increased levels of cytokines and proteases in chronic wounds decrease mitogenic activities and the response of wound cells, thus impairing healing.[54]

DISCLOSURE

S.R. Goldberg: Investigative PI for Pfizer and UCB studies. R.F. Diegelmann: No Disclosures.

REFERENCES

1. Diegelmann RF, Evans MC. Wound healing: an overview of acute, fibrotic and delayed healing. Front Biosci 2004;9:283–9.
2. Lazarus GS, Cooper DM, Knighton DR, et al. Definitions and guidelines for assessment of wounds and evaluation of healing. Arch Dermatol 1994;130: 489–93.
3. Demidova-Rice TN, Hamblin MR, Herman IM. Acute and impaired wound healing: pathophysiology and current methods for drug delivery, part 1: normal and chronic wounds: biology, causes, and approaches to care. Adv Skin Wound Care 2012;25(7):304–14.

4. Eming SA, Martin P, Tomic-Canic M. Wound repair and regeneration: mechanisms, signaling, and translation. Sci Transl Med 2014;6(265):265sr6.
5. Edwards GA, Shymanska NV, Pierce JG. 5-Benzylidene-4-oxazolidinones potently inhibit biofilm formation in Methicillin-resistant Staphylococcus aureus. Chem Commun (Camb) 2017;53(53):7353–6.
6. Wolcott RD. Biofilms cause chronic infections. J Wound Care 2017;26(8):423–5.
7. Zhao R, Liang H, Clarke E, et al. Inflammation in Chronic Wounds. Int J Mol Sci 2016;17(12). https://doi.org/10.3390/ijms17122085.
8. Pardes JB, Takagi H, Martin TA, et al. Decreased levels of alpha 1(I) procollagen mRNA in dermal fibroblasts grown on fibrin gels and in response to fibrinopeptide B. J Cell Physiol 1995;162(1):9–14.
9. Rajendran S, Rigby AJ, Anand SC. Venous leg ulcer treatment and practice–part 1: the causes and diagnosis of venous leg ulcers. J Wound Care 2007; 16(1):24–6.
10. Frank PG, Lisanti MP. ICAM-1: role in inflammation and in the regulation of vascular permeability. Am J Physiol Heart Circ Physiol 2008;295(3):H926–7.
11. Donohue CM, Adler JV, Bolton LL. Peripheral arterial disease screening and diagnostic practice: a scoping review. Int Wound J 2019. https://doi.org/10.1111/iwj.13223.
12. Steinberg JP, Gurjala AN, Jia S, et al. Evaluating the effects of subclinical, cyclic ischemia-reperfusion injury on wound healing using a novel device in the rabbit ear. Ann Plast Surg 2014;72(6):698–705.
13. Diegelmann RF. Excessive neutrophils characterize chronic pressure ulcers. Wound Repair Regen 2003;11(6):490–5.
14. Nickinson ATO, Bridgwood B, Houghton JSM, et al. A systematic review investigating the identification, causes, and outcomes of delays in the management of chronic limb-threatening ischemia and diabetic foot ulceration. J Vasc Surg 2019. https://doi.org/10.1016/j.jvs.2019.08.229.
15. Dinh T, Scovell S, Veves A. Peripheral arterial disease and diabetes: a clinical update. Int J Low Extrem Wounds 2009;8(2):75–81.
16. Jhamb S, Vangaveti VN, Malabu UH. Genetic and molecular basis of diabetic foot ulcers: clinical review. J Tissue Viability 2016;25(4):229–36.
17. Braun LR, Fisk WA, Lev-Tov H, et al. Diabetic foot ulcer: an evidence-based treatment update. Am J Clin Dermatol 2014;15(3):267–81.
18. Galkowska H, Wojewodzka U, Olszewski WL. Chemokines, cytokines, and growth factors in keratinocytes and dermal endothelial cells in the margin of chronic diabetic foot ulcers. Wound Repair Regen 2006;14(5):558–65.
19. Lobmann R, Ambrosch A, Schultz G, et al. Expression of matrix-metalloproteinases and their inhibitors in the wounds of diabetic and non-diabetic patients. Diabetologia 2002;45(7):1011–6.
20. Cho J, Mosher DF. Role of fibronectin assembly in platelet thrombus formation. J Thromb Haemost 2006;4(7):1461–9.
21. Rabhi-Sabile S, de Romeuf C, Pidard D. On the mechanism of plasmin-induced aggregation of human platelets: implication of secreted von Willebrand factor. Thromb Haemost 1998;79(6):1191–8.
22. Ono Y, Kurano M, Ohkawa R, et al. Sphingosine 1-phosphate release from platelets during clot formation: close correlation between platelet count and serum sphingosine 1-phosphate concentration. Lipids Health Dis 2013;12:20.
23. Gailit J, Clark RA. Wound repair in the context of extracellular matrix. Curr Opin Cell Biol 1994;6(5):717–25.

24. Diegelmann RF, Cohen IK, Kaplan AM. The role of macrophages in wound repair: a review. Plast Reconstr Surg 1981;68(1):107–13.
25. Ribatti D, Tamma R. Giulio Gabbiani and the discovery of myofibroblasts. Inflamm Res 2019;68(3):241–5.
26. Krishnaswamy VR, Mintz D, Sagi I. Matrix metalloproteinases: the sculptors of chronic cutaneous wounds. Biochim Biophys Acta Mol Cell Res 2017;1864(11 Pt B):2220–7.
27. Vaalamo M, Leivo T, Saarialho-Kere U. Differential expression of tissue inhibitors of metalloproteinases (TIMP-1, -2, -3, and -4) in normal and aberrant wound healing. Hum Pathol 1999;30(7):795–802.
28. Clore JN, Cohen IK, Diegelmann RF. Quantitation of collagen types I and III during wound healing in rat skin. Proc Soc Exp Biol Med 1979;161(3):337–40.
29. Frykberg RG, Banks J. Challenges in the Treatment of Chronic Wounds. Adv Wound Care (New Rochelle) 2015;4(9):560–82.
30. Tipton CD, Mathew ME, Wolcott RA, et al. Temporal dynamics of relative abundances and bacterial succession in chronic wound communities. Wound Repair Regen 2017;25(4):673–9.
31. Wolcott RD, Hanson JD, Rees EJ, et al. Analysis of the chronic wound microbiota of 2,963 patients by 16S rDNA pyrosequencing. Wound Repair Regen 2016; 24(1):163–74.
32. Gallo RL. S. epidermidis influence on host immunity: more than skin deep. Cell Host Microbe 2015;17(2):143–4.
33. Scharschmidt TC, Fischbach MA. What lives on our skin: ecology, genomics and therapeutic opportunities of the skin microbiome. Drug Discov Today Dis Mech 2013;10(3–4). https://doi.org/10.1016/j.ddmec.2012.12.003.
34. Leid JG, Willson CJ, Shirtliff ME, et al. The exopolysaccharide alginate protects Pseudomonas aeruginosa biofilm bacteria from IFN-gamma-mediated macrophage killing. J Immunol 2005;175(11):7512–8.
35. Peterson LR. Squeezing the antibiotic balloon: the impact of antimicrobial classes on emerging resistance. Clin Microbiol Infect 2005;11(Suppl 5):4–16.
36. James GA, Swogger E, Wolcott R, et al. Biofilms in chronic wounds. Wound Repair Regen 2008;16(1):37–44.
37. Wolcott RD, Rhoads DD, Dowd SE. Biofilms and chronic wound inflammation. J Wound Care 2008;17(8):333–41.
38. Page-McCaw A, Ewald AJ, Werb Z. Matrix metalloproteinases and the regulation of tissue remodelling. Nat Rev Mol Cell Biol 2007;8(3):221–33.
39. Yan C, Boyd DD. Regulation of matrix metalloproteinase gene expression. J Cell Physiol 2007;211(1):19–26.
40. Pilcher BK, Dumin JA, Sudbeck BD, et al. The activity of collagenase-1 is required for keratinocyte migration on a type I collagen matrix. J Cell Biol 1997; 137(6):1445–57.
41. Yager DR, Zhang LY, Liang HX, et al. Wound fluids from human pressure ulcers contain elevated matrix metalloproteinase levels and activity compared to surgical wound fluids. J Invest Dermatol 1996;107(5):743–8.
42. Grinnell F, Zhu M. Fibronectin degradation in chronic wounds depends on the relative levels of elastase, alpha1-proteinase inhibitor, and alpha2-macroglobulin. J Invest Dermatol 1996;106(2):335–41.
43. Rao CN, Ladin DA, Liu YY, et al. Alpha 1-antitrypsin is degraded and nonfunctional in chronic wounds but intact and functional in acute wounds: the inhibitor protects fibronectin from degradation by chronic wound fluid enzymes. J Invest Dermatol 1995;105(4):572–8.

44. Bickel M. The role of interleukin-8 in inflammation and mechanisms of regulation. J Periodontol 1993;64(5 Suppl):456–60.
45. Mateo RB, Reichner JS, Albina JE. Interleukin-6 activity in wounds. Am J Physiol 1994;266(6 Pt 2):R1840–4.
46. Tanaka T, Narazaki M, Kishimoto T. IL-6 in Inflammation, Immunity, and Disease. Cold Spring Harb Perspect Biol 2014;6(10).
47. Ambrosch A, Lobmann R, Pott A, et al. Interleukin-6 concentrations in wound fluids rather than serological markers are useful in assessing bacterial triggers of ulcer inflammation. Int Wound J 2008;5(1):99–106.
48. Pfeffer K. Biological functions of tumor necrosis factor cytokines and their receptors. Cytokine Growth Factor Rev 2003;14(3–4):185–91.
49. Ashcroft GS, Jeong M-J, Ashworth JJ, et al. Tumor necrosis factor-alpha (TNF-α) is a therapeutic target for impaired cutaneous wound healing. Wound Repair Regen 2012;20(1):38–49.
50. Snyder RJ, Fife C, Moore Z. Components and quality measures of DIME (Devitalized Tissue, Infection/Inflammation, Moisture Balance, and Edge Preparation) in wound care. Adv Skin Wound Care 2016;29(5):205–15.
51. Jones V, Grey JE, Harding KG. Wound dressings. BMJ 2006;332(7544):777–80.
52. Wei D, Zhu X-M, Chen Y-Y, et al. Chronic wound biofilms: diagnosis and therapeutic strategies. Chin Med J 2019. https://doi.org/10.1097/CM9.0000000000000523.
53. Jones RE, Foster DS, Longaker MT. Management of chronic wounds-2018. JAMA 2018;320(14):1481–2.
54. Schultz GS, Chin GA, Moldawer L, et al. Principles of wound healing. In: Fitridge R, Thompson M, editors. Mechanisms of vascular disease: a reference book for vascular specialists. Adelaide (AU): University of Adelaide Press; 2011. p. 423–45. Available at: http://www.ncbi.nlm.nih.gov/books/NBK534261/. Accessed November 25, 2019.

The Effect of Comorbidities on Wound Healing

Robel T. Beyene, MD[a], Stephen Lentz Derryberry Jr, MD[a], Adrian Barbul, MD[a,b,]*

KEYWORDS

- Wound healing • Comorbidities • Delayed wound healing

KEY POINTS

- Wound healing is a complex process that has several steps. Patient comorbidities can interfere with this process.
- Diabetes can inhibit and delay wound healing at several points along the normal process. Other comorbidities may also interfere with wound healing at one or more points.
- External factors (eg, smoking, substance abuse, environmental exposure) and therapeutic modalities can also have a negative effect on wound healing.

INTRODUCTION

Healed wounds represent the final result of a complex and redundant biochemical and cellular process. About 50% of all cases discussed in the weekly morbidity and mortality conferences in departments of surgery around the country reflect a failure of the healing process, either through underresponses and overresponses. Therefore, practicing surgeons should not take the healing process for granted and need be aware of the many factors that affect this important response (**Table 1**).

HERITABLE DISEASES OF CONNECTIVE TISSUE

Genetically determined, primary disorders of connective tissue exist and may involve collagen, elastin, or mucopolysaccharides. The major types, discussed in this article, raise unique challenges to the surgeon.

Ehlers-Danlos Syndrome

Ehlers-Danlos syndrome (EDS) comprises distinct disorders that represent a defect in collagen formation. It is a heterogeneous group of inheritable connective tissue disorders characterized by skin hyperextensibility, joint hypermobility, and cutaneous

[a] Department of Surgery, Vanderbilt University Medical Center, 1310 24th Avenue South, Nashville, TN 37212, USA; [b] Department of Surgery, Nashville Veterans Administration Hospital, 1310 24th Avenue South, Nashville, TN 37212, USA
* Corresponding author. Department of Surgery, Nashville Veterans Administration Hospital, 1310 24th Avenue South, Nashville, TN 37212.
E-mail address: adrian.barbul@vumc.org

Surg Clin N Am 100 (2020) 695–705
https://doi.org/10.1016/j.suc.2020.05.002
0039-6109/20/Published by Elsevier Inc.

Table 1 Factors affecting wound healing	

Genetic	Inborn errors of collagen synthesis
	  Ehlers-Danlos
	  Marfan syndrome
	  Osteogenesis imperfecta
	  Epidermolysis bullosa

Systemic	Metabolic
	  Diabetes mellitus
	  Chronic renal failure
	Nutritional
	  Malnutrition
	  Obesity
	  Vitamin deficiencies
	Cardiovascular
	  Chronic obstructive pulmonary disease
	  Congestive heart failure
	Inflammatory/autoimmune
	  Vasculitis
	  Rheumatoid arthritis
	  Systemic lupus erythematosus
	  Scleroderma
	  Granulomatosis with polyangiitis (previously Wegener)
	  Polyarteritis nodosa
	  Cryoglobulinemia
	  Raynaud disease
	  Pyoderma
	Environmental/toxin
	  Smoking
	  Alcohol
	  Drugs of abuse

Infectious	Bacterial

Post-therapy	Chemotherapy
	Radiation
	Drugs
	  Steroids
	  Nonsteroidal anti-inflammatory drugs

fragility with delayed wound healing. More than half of the affected patients have genetic defects encoding alpha chains of collagen type V, causing it to be either quantitatively or structurally defective. Other subtypes of EDS affect the synthesis and organization of the extracellular matrix through enzymatic defects. The disorders are manifest by thin, friable skin with prominent veins, easy bruising, poor wound healing, atrophic scar formation, recurrent hernias, and hyperextensible joints.[1,2] Gastrointestinal problems include bleeding, hiatal hernia, intestinal diverticula, and rectal prolapse. Small blood vessels are fragile, making suturing difficult during surgery. Large vessels may develop aneurysms, varicosities, arteriovenous fistulas, or may spontaneously rupture.[3]

Recently there has been description of a vascular EDS caused by heterozygous mutations in the COL3A1 gene; this leads to qualitative and quantitative defects of type III collagen, expressed mainly in soft connective tissues and hollow organs, and thus leading to spontaneous artery dissection or rupture, bowel perforation, and pneumothorax.

There is no cure for EDS, and therefore preoperative recognition is vital to optimize management and prevent serious, but possibly avoidable, complications. This syndrome must be considered in every child with recurrent hernias and coagulopathy. Inguinal hernias in these children resemble those seen in adults. Great care should be taken to avoid tearing the skin and fascia; the transversalis fascia is thin and the internal ring is greatly dilated. An adult-type repair with the use of mesh may lower the incidence of recurrence.

In all patients, dermal wounds should be closed in two layers, without tension, and the sutures should be left in place twice as long as usual; additionally, external fixation with adhesive tape can help reinforce the scar and prevent stretching.[3]

Marfan Syndrome

Marfan syndrome is an autosomal-dominant genetic disorder, secondary to mutations in the genes encoding fibrillin-1; the defect in FBN1 gene function leads to increased transforming growth factor-β signaling, particularly in the aortic wall.[4] Excess transforming growth factor-β results in elastin lysis in the media of the vascular wall, increasing the risk of vascular complications. Patients with the syndrome have tall stature, arachnodactyly, lax ligaments, myopia, scoliosis, pectus excavatum, and aneurysm of the ascending aorta. Patients who suffer from this syndrome also are prone to hernias. Surgical repairs of any of these is challenging, because the soft connective tissue fails to hold sutures. Skin is hyperextensible, but shows no delay in wound healing.[3,5]

Osteogenesis Imperfecta

Patients with osteogenesis imperfecta, a mutation in type I collagen, have brittle bones, osteopenia, low muscle mass, hernias, and ligament and joint laxity. Osteogenesis imperfecta subtypes range from mild to lethal manifestations. Patients experience dermal thinning and increased propensity to bruising. Scarring is normal and the skin is not hyperextensible. Surgery is successful but difficult in these patients, because the bones fracture easily under minimal stress.

Epidermolysis Bullosa

Epidermolysis bullosa manifestations include impairment in tissue adhesion within the epidermis, basement membrane, or dermis, resulting in tissue separation and blistering with minimal trauma. The recessively inherited dystrophic type is characterized by defects in the COL7A1 gene, encoding type 7 collagen, important for connecting the epidermis to the dermis, therefore phenotypically resulting in blistering.[6]

Management of nonhealing wounds in patients with epidermolysis bullosa is challenging, because nutritional status is compromised secondary to oral erosions and esophageal obstruction. Surgical interventions include esophageal dilatation and gastrostomy tube placement. Dermal incisions must be meticulously placed to avoid further trauma to skin.[7] Blistering at the postoperative site seems to be uncommon and use of nonadhesive pads covered by "bulky" dressing is recommended. Postoperative wound infections and dehiscence are uncommon, but have a risk for keloid or hypertrophic scarring development.[8]

SYSTEMIC FACTORS
Metabolic

Diabetes mellitus
Diabetes is a growing, worldwide disease that will affect 40 million people by 2030 and currently costs more than $25 billion worldwide.[9] More than a hundred alterations in

wound healing have been identified in people with diabetes, spanning across all phases of healing.[10] Patients with diabetes show hormonal dysregulation, decreased neuropeptide release, delayed platelet activation, and irregular molecular signaling and release in the hemostatic phase. Diabetes mellitus affects cell migration and activation during the inflammatory phase. Collagen deposition, angiogenesis, epithelialization, and granulation tissue formation, all hallmarks of the proliferative phase, are also altered. The maturation phase evinces increase in matrix metalloproteases activity and alterations in collagen turnover.[11]

The systemic changes associated with diabetes have an additive effect in delaying wound healing. These include not only hyperglycemia and peripheral arterial disease, but also worsening renal function, malnutrition, and the high risk of reinjury associated with peripheral neuropathy. Hyperglycemia contributes to enzyme and protein dysfunction, which alters cell and nutrient delivery by affecting basement membranes. Glycation of collagen and other proteins perpetuates the inflammatory alterations in diabetes.[11] Vascular disease contributes to the local tissue hypoxia.[12] Furthermore, the patient with diabetes is prone to infection because of lessened antimicrobial resistance, thus complicating wound healing and increasing the risk of amputation or death.[13]

Another hallmark of diabetic wound healing is perturbation of angiogenesis during the proliferative phase. The balance of proangiogenic and antiangiogenic factors necessary for hemostasis is altered after injury.[11,14] Baseline microvascular and macrovascular disease and hyperglycemia lead to excessive tissue hypoxia at the injury site, further impairing angiogenesis.

Macrophages, normally a source of vascular endothelial growth factor and proangiogenic factors in normal wound healing, are deficient in number and activity in diabetes mellitus, whereas there is a simultaneous upregulation of antiangiogenic factors. The impaired angiogenesis affects downstream granulation and epithelialization functions, and eventually on the maturation phase of the wound.[14]

The classically described chronic diabetic wound is the diabetic foot ulcer: painful, chronic sores with disintegration of overlying tissue, which often involve tendons and bones.[14] Peripheral neuropathy and microvascular changes, and hyperglycemia and peripheral vascular disease, lead to fragile skin and subcutaneous tissue and the development of tissue ischemia and ulceration. Once injured, inflammatory molecules (cytokines and proteases), reactive oxygen species, and senescent cells take root. Persistent infection and a biofilm can also develop.[13] The inflammatory drive, which is present in normal wound healing, becomes persistent and maladaptive, leading to worsening tissue destruction and halting the normal progression of wound healing before the proliferative phase can begin. A cascade of increasing reactive oxygen species, proteases, and inflammatory cytokines makes what might have been an acute injury that heals without intervention into a chronic wound that may progress to limb dysfunction, amputation, or even death.

Failure to restore the skin's natural barrier function is a critical component in turning an acute wound into a chronic wound, or even into a recurrent wound. Even if a patient with diabetes is able to heal a wound, the innate factors of poorly controlled diabetes remain in place and continue to jeopardize the patient's healing. For example, ongoing neuropathy makes the patient less able to protect against exposure to heat, moisture, trauma, or pressure, all of which can reinjure the wound. Similarly, the quality of the healed wound and stability of the tissue layers is diminished.[15]

Appropriate glycemic control can do much to improve acute and chronic wound healing in patients with diabetes. Although this is challenging, it is possible in most patients with diabetes and should be undertaken before elective procedures, aiming for a hemoglobin A_{1c} level of less than eight.[9]

Renal failure

Although chronic kidney disease and end-stage kidney disease occur most often in patients with multiple comorbid conditions, they carry an innate risk of diminished wound healing.[16] After accounting for the contributions of concomitant diabetes, peripheral vascular disease, and aging, kidney disease confers an independent risk of poor wound healing. Acute kidney injury is most commonly associated with severe trauma (especially crush injuries), burns, surgical wounds, and infectious wounds. Given this constellation, it is difficult to identify the contribution of kidney injury alone to healing impairment. Although animal studies have noted inhibition of fibroblast and capillary proliferation in acute kidney injury, these defects are most notable in patients who progress to severe uremia.[17]

Chronic kidney disease affects wound healing through tissue edema, disruption of keratinization kinetics, delayed granulation, and large epithelial gaps. Chronic inflammation, diminished angiogenesis, and cell proliferation also contribute to poor wound healing in chronic kidney disease. Clinical studies have also shown an increase in wound disruption.[16]

Uremia adversely affects fibroblasts, impairs hydroxyproline and collagen formation, and this defect can improve with dialysis or transplantation.[16] Even with dialysis, some molecules too large for removal by dialysis can continue to accumulate to toxic levels causing tissue fragility, platelet dysfunction, impaired hemostasis, continued inflammation, generation of oxygen radicals, and impaired collagen function, all significant roadblocks to wound healing.

Renal dialysis, although life sustaining, contributes to poor wound healing. Unavoidable losses of protein, water-soluble vitamins, and minerals (zinc, selenium, and especially iron), lead to deficiencies that impact normal healing; supplemental, protein, vitamins, and minerals can reverse this process.[16]

There is an elevated risk of infection in patients with end-stage kidney disease and mortality secondary to sepsis is 100- to 300-fold higher in patients undergoing dialysis and 20-fold higher in renal transplant recipients.[18] The mechanism may involve diminished phagocytic function, ischemia, and microcirculatory impairment.[16]

Smoking

The negative effects of cigarette smoking on wound healing have been documented for more than four decades.[19] Inhalation of gaseous (eg, carbon monoxide, hydrogen cyanide) and particulate (nicotine) toxins, which are able to enter the bloodstream, is believed to play a part. Nicotine inhibits red blood cell, fibroblast, and macrophage proliferation, while also causing microclot formation and decreased microperfusion through increased platelet aggregation; cutaneous vasoconstriction with release of catecholamines, which worsen wound ischemia, is also a consequence of nicotine. Carbon monoxide competes for oxygen uptake in red blood cells and decreases wound perfusion, both causing wound hypoxia.

Although smoking enhances platelet activation and fibrin cross-linking in the hemostatic phase, the composition of the clot is abnormal.[20] In the inflammatory phase, smoking increases neutrophil cell count, but depresses chemotactic responsiveness, migration, enzyme release, and bactericidal mechanisms.

Further alterations in smokers involve monocyte migration, macrophage cellularity, increased generation of oxygen radicals, impaired phagocytosis, excessive collagenolysis, and alterations in number of matrix metalloproteases. Overall, delayed wound healing is characteristically present and many elective procedures (eg, hernia repairs, cosmetic, joint replacement) are withheld in smokers.[20] Although data on the effects of vaping are lacking, inhaled gaseous compounds common to vaping and traditional cigarettes likely have similar effects.

Nutrition

Malnutrition

Nutritional deficits make tissue easier to injure and harder to heal.[21] All phases of healing require protein and energy substrates for successful completion.[22] Furthermore, electrolytes, minerals, and vitamins serve as cofactors in the wound healing process, and are all limited in cases of malnutrition.

Even short periods of starvation delay healing (biologic priority of healing wound). As the starvation is prolonged, there is decreased neovascularization and collagen synthesis, prolonged inflammatory phase, decreased phagocytosis, dysfunction of immune cells, and decreased mechanical strength of the repaired tissue. Avoidance of malnutrition is preferable to treating it, but once recognized, it is important to act decisively. Targeted oral nutrient supplementation is postulated to improve healing of wounds in malnourished patients. Protein deficiency can interfere with immune cell function and collagen deposition. Glutamine, arginine, methionine, and cysteine are known to be necessary in wound healing, but only arginine has been shown to be effective following directed supplementation. Arginine is involved in immune, endocrine, and endothelial functions necessary to wound healing and is the precursor to proline, which is pivotal to collagen deposition, angiogenesis, and wound contraction.[22-24] Zinc and iron supplementation is indicated in patients with deficiency in those minerals, but the benefit of supernormal supplementation is unproven.[22]

Fatty acid deficiency limits cell membrane synthesis and can limit normal inflammation necessary to wound healing. Vitamin C (ascorbic acid) is required for proline-lysine hydroxylation and cross-linkage needed to stabilize collagen, and normal immune response and cell mitosis and migration.[22]

Obesity

Complications of wound healing associated with obesity include infection, dehiscence, hematoma and seroma formation, and pressure and venous ulceration.[25] The increased risk of wound infection in obese patients is widely confirmed. The avascular nature of adipose tissue leads to local hypoxia, which impedes neutrophil function and bacterial clearance; delivery of antibiotics to the wound is also impaired.[23] Dehiscence, and hematoma and seroma formation, are traced primarily to mechanical factors, because wounds are under greater tension and obliteration of dead space is more challenging. These factors also increase the risk of infection.

In healthy obese rodents, there is decreased wound mechanical strength and reparative collagen deposition, confirming that even uncomplicated obesity impairs healing (**Fig. 1**).

Aging

Aging causes decreased collagen density, decreased fibroblast numbers, and increased elastin fragmentation in uninjured skin. Past the age of 50, there is a roughly a 1% per year decrease in dermal collagen content. The dermis, a major contributor to cosmesis of skin, loses thickness, elasticity, and water content in aging. Dermal glycosaminoglycans, which are involved in granulation, water binding, and epithelialization, undergo molecular changes. Aged skin also has reduced dermal blood vessels, which limits oxygen and nutrient delivery to the wound. The subcutaneous fat thins in some areas and swells in others over time, which mitigates the thermoregulatory and

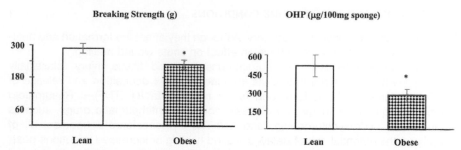

Fig. 1. Wound breaking strength and wound collagen deposition, measure as hydroxyproline (OHP), in subcutaneously implanted sponges in lean and obese Leprfa/Leprfa Zucker rats. * $p<0.05$.[46]

barrier functions of that layer. The tensile strength of skin diminishes, making wound closure slower and less reliable.[26]

Clinically, this means that by 40 years old, the time it takes to heal a wound can double, relative to a 20 year old with an identical wound.[26,27] Epithelial healing, as in donor sites for split-thickness skin grafts, decreases significantly with aging; collagen synthesis in dermis does not appear diminished, but its quality is different.[28] These changes, and the increased incidence of comorbidities, leads to delays in wound healing in aging skin, although this is more evident in chronic wounds than in acute wound healing in healthy, older adults.[26]

Age-related hormone changes, specifically sex hormones, have also been implicated in wound healing delays in elderly men.[23] Estrogen, androgen, and dehydroepiandrosterone gene expression differences lead to variable expression of genes involved sex hormone production. Because elderly women tend to heal wounds better than elderly men, beneficial effects of estrogens and adverse effects of androgens have been implicated.

INFECTIONS

The proper unfolding of wound healing is susceptible to disruption in the presence of infection. Although the exact mechanism by which infection interferes with wound healing is not entirely understood and likely multifactorial, it is thought that the presence of and resultant inflammation delays the proliferative and remodeling stages. The spectrum of influence caused by infection ranges from chronic wound development to tissue necrosis, possible dissemination of infection, sepsis, and ultimately death. Bacteria also produce collagenases, which destroy reparative collagen. There is an increased association between wound infections and postoperative incisional hernia formation and anastomotic failure in the presence of peritoneal infection.

Surgical site infections (SSIs) remain a major source of morbidity and mortality. Treatment standardization of SSIs is difficult given the wide variation of wound location, size, mechanism, age, and offending infectious agent. The implementation of postoperative protocols aimed at decreasing the incidence of SSIs shows little impact on clinical practice but remains a major area of research. Studies comparing the use of specific types of postoperative dressings, timing of dressing removal, resumption of normal bathing habits, the use of postoperative systemic or topical antibiotics for burn wounds and wounds healing by secondary intention, as a means for SSI prevention are inconclusive.[29–33]

INFLAMMATORY AND AUTOIMMUNE CONDITIONS

Diverse diseases comprise this category. Although they affect the formation and healing of chronic wounds, they also have an effect on acute wound healing.

Rheumatoid arthritis leads to autoimmune-mediated tissue injury, classically involving the synovial membranes, via immune complex deposition and release of cytokines interleukin (IL)-1, IL-6, and tumor necrosis factor (TNF)-α. Rheumatoid arthritis is frequently managed by disease-modifying antirheumatic drugs, such as methotrexate, hydroxychloroquine, and anti-TNF-α monoclonal antibodies, all of which have the potential risk of delayed wound healing or increased infections postoperatively. However, most clinical studies do not support an association with delayed wound healing or increased risk of SSI.[34,35]

Vasculitides are disorders characterized by inflammation of the vascular system and include thromboangiitis obliterans (affecting the small- and medium-sized vessels of the hands and feet), polyarteritis nodosa (affecting medium-sized muscular arteries), and Behçet disease (affecting small vessels throughout many regions of the body). The inflammation, subsequent thrombosis, and vessel destruction characteristic of vasculitides disrupts oxygen and nutrient delivery to the healing wound.[36]

Vasculitides can result in necrotic ulcerations and tissue loss, which is difficult to heal. Treatment involves the use of immunosuppressants, such as prednisone and cyclophosphamide. Immunosuppression may result in improvement of wound healing (in chronic wounds), or could impair acute healing.

Scleroderma is a constellation of disorders characterized by abnormal T-lymphocyte activation, ischemic fibrosis, and production of altered connective tissues. Manifestations can include areas of thickened skin, secondary Raynaud phenomenon (arterial spasm affecting the digits), dysphagia, and telangiectasias. Similar to rheumatoid arthritis, women are more commonly affected than men and the disorder tends to manifest in middle age. Immunomodulators (ie, corticosteroids, methotrexate) and symptomatic control are the mainstay of treatment. Chronic ulcerations, especially on digits, are common.

Pyoderma gangrenosum is a rare condition characterized by painful nodules and/ or sterile pustules, which progress to ulcerations. More than 50% of cases are associated with other autoimmune disorders (eg, ulcerative colitis, rheumatoid arthritis). Pyoderma gangrenosum is considered a neutrophilic dermatosis, a group of autoinflammatory skin conditions characterized by a preponderance of neutrophils on histology. The treatment of pyoderma gangrenosum includes topical corticosteroids, anti-inflammatory antibiotics (ie, doxycycline, minocycline), intralesional steroid injections, intravenous immunoglobulin, and other immunomodulators (eg, mycophenolate mofetil, dapsone, azathioprine, TNF-α inhibitors, and other biologics).[37,38]

Systemic lupus erythematosus is a collection of autoimmune disorders characterized by antibodies to specific intracellular components (eg, nuclear proteins, DNA, phospholipid). Immunomodulators, antimalarials, and symptomatic control are the mainstay of treatment. Aberrant IL-2 function is thought to play a key role in the development of the disorder and low-dose administration of IL-2 has been shown to expand regulatory T-cell function, resulting in a decrease in autoimmune activity.[39]

All of these disorders can affect wound healing and their respective therapy often can negatively affect acute healing.

CANCER THERAPY
Chemotherapy

Because of characteristic accelerated cell turnover, fresh wounds are susceptible to growth inhibition by antineoplastic agents. Most such agents interfere with DNA or

RNA replication, protein synthesis, or cell division and thus directly affect the proliferative phase of wound healing by inhibiting fibroplasia, angiogenesis, and epithelialization. Less agents affect wound strength during the remodeling phase.

Knowledge of interference of chemotherapy with wound healing is mainly based on animal studies. Usually, doses of chemotherapeutic agents in different animal species and humans are comparable when the dose is measured in milligram per square meter of surface area.[23] Assuming that these findings are applicable to humans, the results vary according to drug class, the time of administration relative to wounding, the dose of drug, and the time period between surgery and subsequent investigation of wound parameters. Although alkylating agents, antimetabolites, plant alkaloids, and antitumor antibiotics have different mechanisms of action, their effect on wounds seems limited to the proliferative phase, but no typical impairment patterns have been found according to drug class; additionally, most antineoplastic agents also have systemic effects, such as weight loss, leukopenia, and anemia, which affect wound responses. Usually only high or therapeutic dosages affect healing.

Most human studies do not document increases in wound complication rates from use of chemotherapeutic agents. Delaying start of such regimens for 7 to 10 days postoperatively impacts minimally on wound healing.

Corticosteroids are frequently used in patients with cancer; they are well-known inhibitors of the inflammatory response and subsequent fibroplasia, and these effects are noted following either acute or long-term use. Delay of steroid use for the first 5 days postoperatively and/or the use of vitamin A abrogated the negative effects on wounds.[40–42]

Radiotherapy

Patients undergoing surgery for tumor treatment often receive combined radiotherapy and chemotherapy. Preoperative or early postoperative radiation negatively impacts wound healing. Concomitant use of radiotherapy and chemotherapy seems to have additive negative affect on wounds.

Radiated tissue heals poorly resulting in increased rate of fistulas, wound necrosis, delayed healing, flap failures, and infection.[43] The longer the interval from the administration of radiation, the stronger the impact on wound healing. Irradiated tissue is hypoxic because of fibrosis of capillary and small-caliber vessels.[44]

Preoperative radiotherapy is frequently used in modern cancer care and surgical interventions are carried out 4 to 8 weeks after the end of the treatment. Doses larger than 50 Gy result in increased wound complications.[45] The negative effects of radiation continue throughout the life of the patient and late interventions on radiated bowel or soft tissue is fraught with complications.

SUMMARY

This article highlights many of the conditions or therapies that can adversely affect wounds. Planning for surgical interventions requires an awareness of such preexisting conditions. The surgeon should exercise care and approach such wounds with caution, including use of permanent rather than absorbable sutures; maintaining skin closure for longer than usual; proper antibiotic prophylaxis; and if time permits, correction of nutritional deficits.

DISCLOSURE

The authors have nothing to disclose.

REFERENCES

1. Phillips C, Wenstrup RJ. Biosynthetic and genetic disorders of collagen. In: Cohen K, Diegelman R, Winbald W, editors. Wound healing, biochemical and clinical. Philadelphia: WB Saunders Co; 1992. p. 254–61.
2. Sidhu-Malik NK, Wenstrup RJ. The Ehlers-Danlos syndromes and Marfan syndrome: inherited diseases of connective tissue with overlapping clinical features. Semin Dermatol 1995;14(1):40–6.
3. Malfait F, Wenstrup RJ, De Paepe A. Clinical and genetic aspects of Ehlers-Danlos syndrome, classic type. Genet Med 2010;12(10):597–605.
4. Wagner AH, Zaradzki M, Arif R, et al. Marfan syndrome: a therapeutic challenge for long-term care. Biochem Pharmacol 2019;164:53–63.
5. Hunt TK. Disorders of wound healing. World J Surg 1980;4(3):271–7.
6. Knaup J, Verwanger T, Gruber C, et al. Epidermolysis bullosa: a group of skin diseases with different causes but commonalities in gene expression. Exp Dermatol 2012;21(7):526–30.
7. Carter DM, Lin AN. Wound healing and epidermolysis bullosa. Arch Dermatol 1988;124(5):732–3.
8. Harris AG, Saikal SL, Murrell DF. Epidermolysis bullosa patients' perception of surgical wound and scar healing. Dermatol Surg 2019;45(2):280–9.
9. Han G, Ceilley R. Chronic wound healing: a review of current management and treatments. Adv Ther 2017;34(3):599–610.
10. Brem H, Tomic-Canic M. Cellular and molecular basis of wound healing in diabetes. J Clin Invest 2007;117(5):1219–22.
11. Baltzis D, Eleftheriadou I, Veves A. Pathogenesis and treatment of impaired wound healing in diabetes mellitus: new insights. Adv Ther 2014;31(8):817–36.
12. Janis JE, Harrison B. Wound healing: part I. Basic science. Plast Reconstr Surg 2014;133(2):199e–207e.
13. Frykberg RG, Banks J. Challenges in the treatment of chronic wounds. Adv Wound Care 2015;4(9):560–82.
14. Okonkwo UA, DiPietro LA. Diabetes and wound angiogenesis. Int J Mol Sci 2017;18(7).
15. Sorg H, Tilkorn DJ, Hager S, et al. Skin wound healing: an update on the current knowledge and concepts. Eur Surg Res 2017;58(1–2):81–94.
16. Maroz N, Simman R. Wound healing in patients with impaired kidney function. J Am Coll Clin Wound Spec 2013;5(1):2–7.
17. McDermott FT, Nayman J, De Boer WG. The effect of acute renal failure upon wound healing: histological and autoradiographic studies in the mouse. Ann Surg 1968;168(1):142–6.
18. Sarnak MJ, Jaber BL. Mortality caused by sepsis in patients with end-stage renal disease compared with the general population. Kidney Int 2000;58(4):1758–64.
19. Silverstein P. Smoking and wound healing. Am J Med 1992;93(1A):22S–4S.
20. Sorensen LT. Wound healing and infection in surgery: the pathophysiological impact of smoking, smoking cessation, and nicotine replacement therapy: a systematic review. Ann Surg 2012;255(6):1069–79.
21. Winkler MF, Makowski S. Wound healing. In: Touger-Decker R, Mobley C, Epstein JB, editors. Nutrition and oral medicine. 2nd edition. New York: Springer; 2005. p. 273–81.
22. Wild T, Rahbarnia A, Kellner M, et al. Basics in nutrition and wound healing. Nutrition 2010;26(9):862–6.
23. Guo S, Dipietro LA. Factors affecting wound healing. J Dent Res 2010;89(3):219–29.

24. Chow O, Barbul A. Immunonutrition: role in wound healing and tissue regeneration. Adv Wound Care (New Rochelle) 2014;3(1):46–53.
25. Wilson JA, Clark JJ. Obesity: impediment to postsurgical wound healing. Adv Skin Wound Care 2004;17(8):426–35.
26. Thomas DR, Burkemper NM. Aging skin and wound healing. Clin Geriatr Med 2013;29(2):xi–xx.
27. Gantwerker EA, Hom DB. Skin: histology and physiology of wound healing. Facial Plast Surg Clin North Am 2011;19(3):441–53.
28. Holt DR, Kirk SJ, Regan MC, et al. Effect of age on wound healing in healthy human beings. Surgery 1992;112(2):293–7 [discussion: 297–8].
29. Dumville JC, Gray TA, Walter CJ, et al. Dressings for the prevention of surgical site infection. Cochrane Database Syst Rev 2016;(12):CD003091.
30. Heal CF, Banks JL, Lepper PD, et al. Topical antibiotics for preventing surgical site infection in wounds healing by primary intention. Cochrane Database Syst Rev 2016;(11):CD011426.
31. Norman G, Dumville JC, Mohapatra DP, et al. Antibiotics and antiseptics for surgical wounds healing by secondary intention. Cochrane Database Syst Rev 2016;(3):CD011712.
32. Barajas-Nava LA, Lopez-Alcalde J, Roque i Figuls M, et al. Antibiotic prophylaxis for preventing burn wound infection. Cochrane Database Syst Rev 2013;(6):CD008738.
33. Toon CD, Lusuku C, Ramamoorthy R, et al. Early versus delayed dressing removal after primary closure of clean and clean-contaminated surgical wounds. Cochrane Database Syst Rev 2015;(9):CD010259.
34. Ishie S, Ito H, Azukizawa M, et al. Delayed wound healing after forefoot surgery in patients with rheumatoid arthritis. Mod Rheumatol 2015;25(3):367–72.
35. Yano K, Ikari K, Takatsuki Y, et al. Longer operative time is the risk for delayed wound healing after forefoot surgery in patients with rheumatoid arthritis. Mod Rheumatol 2016;26(2):211–5.
36. Shanmugam VK. Vasculitic diseases and prothrombotic states contributing to delayed healing in chronic wounds. Curr Dermatol Rep 2016;5(4):270–7.
37. Song H, Lahood N, Mostaghimi A. Intravenous immunoglobulin as adjunct therapy for refractory pyoderma gangrenosum: systematic review of cases and case series. Br J Dermatol 2018;178(2):363–8.
38. Ormerod AD, Thomas KS, Craig FE, et al. Comparison of the two most commonly used treatments for pyoderma gangrenosum: results of the STOP GAP randomised controlled trial. BMJ 2015;350:h2958.
39. Mizui M, Tsokos GC. Low-dose IL-2 in the treatment of lupus. Curr Rheumatol Rep 2016;18(11):68.
40. Ehrlich HP, Hunt TK. Effects of cortisone and vitamin A on wound healing. Ann Surg 1968;167(3):324–8.
41. Oxlund H, Fogdestam I, Viidik A. The influence of cortisol on wound healing of the skin and distant connective tissue response. Surg Gynecol Obstet 1979;148(6):876–80.
42. Green JP. Steroid therapy and wound healing in surgical patients. Br J Surg 1965; 52:523–5.
43. Luce EA. The irradiated wound. Surg Clin North Am 1984;64(4):821–9.
44. Payne WG, Walusimbi MS, Blue ML, et al. Radiated groin wounds: pitfalls in reconstruction. Am Surg 2003;69(11):994–7.
45. Mendelsohn FA, Divino CM, Reis ED, et al. Wound care after radiation therapy. Adv Skin Wound Care 2002;15(5):216–24.
46. Uzgare A, Harlan R, Barbul A. Impairment of wound healing in uncomplicated obesity. Wound Rep Regen 17:A41, #130, 2009.

Foot and Ankle Surgery for Chronic Nonhealing Wounds

Christopher Bibbo, DO[a,b,c,]*, Brittany E. Mayer, DPM[d], Laura A. Michetti, DPM[e]

KEYWORDS

- Wounds • Orthotics • Prosthetics • Surgery • External fixation • Plastic surgery
- Charcot

KEY POINTS

- The etiology of chronic wounds may stem from a variety of disorders, such as Charcot neuroarthropathy, trauma, and congenital and acquired neuromuscular disorders.
- Chronic wounds often are associated with tendon imbalances and bony uniplanar and multiplanar deformities.
- Soft orthotic inserts and braces are utilized for simple off-loading of wounds in the preoperative and postoperative settings.
- Surgical intervention ranges from simple resection of a bony prominence to complex correction, flaps, and off-loading external fixation.
- External fixation allows immediate patient mobilization and full weight bearing for reconstructions as well as major amputations.

Chronic wounds are a challenge for reconstructive orthopedic surgeons. Surgeons must understand orthopedic and plastic surgery techniques as well wound care principles. This emerging discipline was described by L. Scott Levin, as the "orthoplastic" surgeon (ref). This orthoplastic approach consists not only of bone and soft tissue techniques but also the art of off-loading the surgical reconstructive site. Reconstruction of the musculoskeletal system must consider the effects of bone, ligamentous,

[a] Foot and Ankle Surgery, Limb Salvage, Rubin Institute for Advanced Orthopedics, International Center for Limb Lengthening, Sinai Hospital of Baltimore, 2401 West Belvidere Avenue, Baltimore, MD 21215, USA; [b] Reconstructive Plastic and Microsurgery, Rubin Institute for Advanced Orthopedics, International Center for Limb Lengthening, Sinai Hospital of Baltimore, 2401 West Belvidere Avenue, Baltimore, MD 21215, USA; [c] Orthopaedic Trauma, Musculoskeletal Infections, Rubin Institute for Advanced Orthopedics, International Center for Limb Lengthening, Sinai Hospital of Baltimore, 2401 West Belvidere Avenue, Baltimore, MD 21215, USA; [d] Rubin Institute for Advanced Orthopedics, International Center for Limb Lengthening, Sinai Hospital of Baltimore, 2401 West Belvidere Avenue, Baltimore, MD 21215, USA; [e] Veterans Affairs Maryland Healthcare System, Rubin Institute for Advanced Orthopedics, International Center for Limb Lengthening, Sinai Hospital of Baltimore, 2401 West Belvidere Avenue, Baltimore, MD 21215, USA
* Corresponding author.
E-mail address: cbibbo@lifebridgehealth.org

Surg Clin N Am 100 (2020) 707–725
https://doi.org/10.1016/j.suc.2020.05.003
surgical.theclinics.com

and tendinous deforming forces. The orthoplastic approach has a soft tissue reconstructive ladder and a reconstructive elevator, an approach that bypasses lesser, more conservative care plans. Host status and multiple skin-based pathologies also influence the selection of reconstructive techniques.

BONE CONSIDERATIONS

The deforming force of mechanical malalignment, the deforming forces induced by the musculotendinous structures, and laxity of ligamentous structures are the main sources in bone architecture that create abnormal focal pressure points. In neuropathic patients, these factors lead to the development of chronic wounds. There also are posttraumatic, neuromuscular, and congenital causes of chronic wounds. Non-neuropathic bone deformity may stem from trauma, acquired and congenital limb deformities, and the spectrum of poorly fitting appliances (orthotics), such as shoes, inserts, boots, and amputation prosthetics. These bone deformities resulting in chronic wounds dictate the technique and its timing when there is draining sinus, abscess, or osteomyelitis.

Osteomyelitis

Osteomyelitis must be addressed with surgical débridement, intravenous antibiotics, and monitoring response to treatment. Bone débridement must be aggressive and frequent, which often influences the selection of the surgical techniques best suited to meet reconstructive goals. Repeat bone débridement with cultures of all biologic tissues (eg, bone and scar) as well as metal and antibiotic delivery device (eg, antibiotic-impregnated polymethylmethacrylate) should be every 2 weeks to 4 weeks until the bone infection is cleared.

Ideally, antibiotic therapy is based on deep bone cultures, but superficial cultures still can be useful when deep cultures are not clinically available. Osteomyelitis is a complex disease, due to biofilm, cellular senescence, and re-emergence of bacterial infection by quorum sensing. Bacterial pathogens may either incorporate into an existing biofilm or initiate a pathogen-based de novo biofilm (eg, on orthopedic implants).[1,2] Biofilms also accrue necrotic bone and dying osteocytes.[3–7] The presence of quiescent pathologic bacteria (persisters) may activate with the recrudescence of the original infecting organism or the presentation of a new species of pathogen.[2]

This activation of quiescent bacteria, many of which are out of the reproductive phase, often results in negative cultures, hence the utility of 16S polymerase chain reaction. Activation of these bacteria is based on the concept of quorum sensing, a mechanism in which bacteria signal the activation of growth and reproduction by both intraspecies and interspecies cross-talk.[8,9] Long-term antibiotic administration is required for the eradication of bone infection, with the understanding that fungal osteomyelitis may develop. The adverse effects of antibiotic therapy must be monitored with protocols that assess renal, hepatic, hematologic, gastrointestinal, and cochlear-vestibular functions. C-reactive protein and erythrocyte sedimentation rate measurements are useful to monitor the response to therapy.

Bone Architecture

All reconstructive techniques must include an evaluation of changes in the mechanical axis of the limb. Changes in adjacent motion segments, especially with bone loss, need to be noted because these are factors in the creation of abnormal biomechanics, joint instability, and subsequent development of ulceration and its inherent sequelae. Osteoporotic bone may fail more easily when resected for chronic wounds; this necessitates modifications to the surgical approach. Charcot neuroarthropathy results in neurohumoral-mediated bone destruction secondary to alterations in the fine balance of osteogenesis, and osteolysis may result in severe collapse of normal bone architecture, especially in the periarticular areas of the foot. Bone loss from infection or trauma is inherently unstable. All these abnormalities in bone architecture may result in changes in the mechanical axis of the lower extremity, producing an unstable limb.

SOFT TISSUE ENVELOPE, NEUROVASCULAR STATUS, AND EDEMA CONTROL

The soft tissue envelope (STE) is critical to the resolution of chronic wounds. This includes the periwound tissue. Adjacent tissue must be healthy enough to allow flap elevation closure of the donor site and the wound bed. These reconstructive techniques are indispensable when Charcot neuroarthropathy, trauma, neuromuscular disorders, and congenital defects result in deformity and high-pressure points of chronic wounds.

The quality of the periwound tissue is influenced by

- Arterial inflow, to heal a surgical reconstruction, and venous outflow, which may prohibit placement of incisions in certain areas.
- Neurologic status—in neuropathic patients, the propensity to form plantar ulcers influences the choice of technique. These patients also are at risk for the development of neuropathic fractures and dislocations (Charcot foot). These may be best addressed by simple exostectomy and gastrocnemius-soleus release. The most challenging reconstruction may require fusions and volumetric reduction of the involved and adjacent bone.
- Edema—the presence of edema makes the healing of any tissue a challenge; this includes the chronic wound, adjacent flaps, and donor sites.

SPECIFIC SURGICAL TECHNIQUES
Tendon Releases

All surgical procedures require that patients fulfill appropriate vascular and orthopedic selection criteria. Patients often have an acquired equinus deformity that places additional undue forces on forefoot and midfoot wounds. Equinus deformity must be addressed at surgery by gastrocnemius recession and percutaneous or open Achilles tendon lengthening.

Digital tenotomies are utilized for dorsal and acral toe ulcerations. Both toe flexor and extensor tenotomies are performed for ulcers of the dorsum of the toes over the interphalangeal joints. When tenotomies of the toes are contemplated, dorsal extensor toe tenotomies may be performed percutaneously in the office. Supple toe deformities respond to metatarsophalangeal capsulotomies. Fixed digital contractures require full extensor and flexor tenotomies, joint capsule release, and pinning.

In a sequential fashion, if the toe does not straighten, a plantar tenotomy may be done at the digital sulcus or under the proximal interphalangeal joint. If the toe still does not straighten, a metatarsophalangeal capsulotomy is performed. If the toe continues to resist attempts to straighten, then a resection arthroplasty with pinning of the toe is required, which requires a formal operative setting.

The Achilles tendon, comprised of the aponeurosis of the gastrocnemius and soleus, is a powerful deforming force in the sagittal plane, creating concentrated forces on the forefoot and midfoot that contribute to ulceration, especially in Charcot neuroarthropathy (**Fig. 1**A). Long-standing valgus and varus foot deformities and deformities after midfoot amputations[10,11] may be maintained by tendon imbalance and

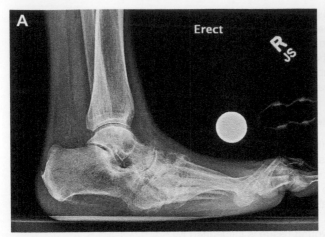
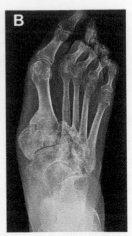

Fig. 1. (*A*) Lateral-view radiograph shows a mild rocker-bottom foot. Note the pressure area at the apex of the plantar deformity. This particular deformity is suitable for an exostectomy and bracing. (*B*) Anteroposterior-view radiograph shows prominence along the medial border of the foot. Often the deformity is planed down and then braced. (Copyright 2020, Rubin Institute for Advanced Orthopedics, Sinai Hospital of Baltimore.)

contribute to chronic medial and lateral wounds, respectively. Release of the deforming tendon or proximal aponeurosis may mitigate this pathologic force. Percutaneous releases may be performed in the office or in the operating room. In diabetics, Achilles tendon lengthening must be performed in 3 locations, with a minimum of 2 cm between tendon cuts. Dorsiflexion should be limited to achieving 5° of dorsiflexion. These rules help decrease the incidence of tendon rupture after lengthening in diabetics and patients who are taking steroids or fluoroquinolones.

Simple Exostectomy

Removal of an area of bony prominence that underlies a chronic wound helps eliminate a source of concentrated pressure. These sites may be anywhere in the foot or ankle. Considerations prior to performing an exostectomy are as follows:

1. Will a tendon insertion be disrupted that results in biomechanical imbalance? An example is disruption of the peroneus brevis tendon.
2. Will the exostectomy result in joint instability? An example is the plantar midfoot in Charcot deformities (see **Fig. 1**A).

The above technique is simple and a good choice for surgeons of all disciplines. Adequate bone resection is mandatory, because inadequate bone resection and failure to assess for the presence of equinus deformity force by the gastrocnemius-soleus complex result in failure. In some cases, just a gastrocnemius-soleus lengthening procedure can provide enough off-loading to heal a wound with local care alone.

Simple Exostectomy with Local Tissue Rearrangements

After exostectomy, a residual wound may exist. The wound may be excised to fresh tissue; then a local skin advancement flap or rotation flap may be performed to achieve wound closure. Local muscle transposition or rotation can be performed followed by human skin substitute application or skin grafting. On the plantar foot, a full-thickness skin graft is preferred, whereas on the non–weight-bearing areas, split-thickness skin grafts are tolerated.

Resection Ostectomy with Deformity Correction

Encompassing a broad array of procedures, resection ostectomy with deformity reconstruction is a powerful approach to reducing wound sites and often eliminates wounds acutely. Single or multiple osteotomies allow for correction of mechanical malalignment of the foot and ankle. A stable foot remains a mainstay in the orthoplastic approach to chronic wounds recalcitrant to conservative measures (**Fig. 1B**). Resection ostectomy with deformity reconstruction requires specialty training, even among experienced orthoplastic and orthopedic surgeons. Fixation of the bone is performed via external fixation, and percutaneous or open stabilization is achieved by utilizing a variety of orthopedic implants.

Reduction Osteoplasty

First described by Bibbo and Stough,[12] reduction osteoplasty is a change in the cubic (volumetric) content of a bone. By doing so, a wound may be excised and primarily closed if the local environment has been converted to a healthy acute wound environment. Reduction osteoplasty also assists with any ancillary soft tissue reconstructive needs for wound coverage. Reduction osteoplasty may be useful particularly when chronic wounds are associated with underlying osteomyelitis, an unstable joint, or tendon imbalance. The procedure may be performed within a bone segment or across a joint, which also may facilitate arthrodesis. Generally, monolateral or circular external fixation is used to facilitate bone healing; the circular external fixator allows early weight-bearing mobilization. Postoperatively, patients must be non–weight bearing until evidence of bone consolidation, followed by an off-loading, diabetic padded ankle-foot orthosis (AFO). Plantar wounds, especially when infected with necrotic tissue, often require multiple débridements, often resulting in a large central defect of the foot. By resecting a central ray, the wound edges may be closed acutely with the use of a miniature external fixator.[13] (please clarify)

Soft Tissue Procedures

Skin grafts often are used in the management of chronic wounds but only after appropriate débridement and management of associated infections. Full-thickness skin grafts are indicated over areas of high-contact shear pressure in nonplantar regions, such as the malleoli. Plantar skin grafts need off-loading, which may be done by implementing a non–weight-bearing status or off-loading orthotics. When a patient is physically able to walk with both limbs, then an off-loading external fixator may be applied, allowing immediate weight bearing while off-loading (floating) the foot off the ground (**Fig. 2**).

Local flaps are invaluable to maintaining Gillies' principle of coverage using "like tissue to cover like tissue." This is important especially on the plantar foot, because the skin and fat pad are highly specialized in this area for pressure tolerance.

After correction of the bony architecture and tendon-induced deforming forces, flaps, such as the V-Y, rotation, and rhomboid, are excellent choices for smaller defects; off-loading is essential for plantar flaps to heal.

The plantar heel is especially difficult to reconstruct. After resection of portions of the calcaneus, if the plantar medial artery (PMA) is patent, the PMA flap is an excellent choice to cover large heel defects. The PMA flap can provide fill of intermediate-depth defects and resurfacing of the STE. When deep defects are present, the abductor hallucis muscle flap and short toe flexor flaps fill the dead space, followed by resurfacing with the PMA flap.

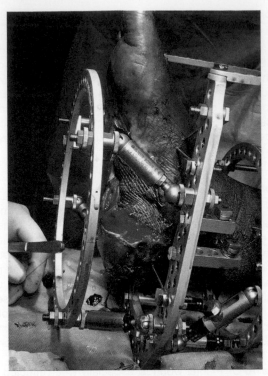

Fig. 2. PMA flap with skin graft and residual wound. This external fixator construct provides off-loading and weight bearing. It is helpful particularly when the time required for healing is prolonged. (Copyright 2020, Dr. Christopher Bibbo, FACS/Main Street Enterprises-Globus Medical, LLC.)

The reverse sural flap is a utilitarian flap for chronic posterior heel wounds. This flap is easily raised, allows for delayed inset in medically compromised patients, and generally has a manageable donor site. The reverse sural flap is a secondary choice for plantar wounds when the PMA flap is not available.

The distally based reverse peroneus brevis muscle flap is an excellent muscle or myocutaneous flap for coverage of chronic lateral ankle and calcaneal wounds.

The combination of flaps with bone resection and off-loading is invaluable in complex wounds.

Small chronic lateral wounds may be covered by the abductor digiti minimi (quinti) (AbdM-5) muscle flap. The AbdM-5 flap is limited due to the small size of the muscle and the complication of lateral column pain resulting from the loss of padding that this muscle provides to the fifth metatarsal. As a result, new chronic wounds may develop that are more difficult to manage than the original wound.

Muscle-Bone Flaps

In instances of a chronic wound débridement resulting in ankle and rearfoot defects with bone loss, the recently developed distally based reverse peroneus brevis-fibula (Rev PB-fib) flap provides wound coverage as well as vascularized bone. (ref) The Rev PB-fib flap is valuable in that it does not interfere with other staged flap procedures. Likewise, a distally based reverse flexor hallucis-fibula flap may be used for chronic soft tissue wounds with a need for bone grafting for chronic wounds of the anterior ankle (ref).

Free flaps are a final consideration for chronic wounds not amenable to local tissue flaps. A prime example is the use of an anterior lateral thigh flap for resulting massive foot defects after wide débridement of the unstable STE with or without osteomyelitis.

NONSURGICAL INTERVENTIONS: OFF-LOADING AND BRACING TO ASSIST WITH HEALING OF CHRONIC WOUNDS OF THE FOOT AND ANKLE

Off-loading shoe gear, inserts, and bracing are important components of the overall treatment plan for chronic wounds, used in settings of both nonoperative management and the perioperative period for surgical reconstructions. Patients with diabetic peripheral neuropathy require special off-loading to prevent recurrent ulcerations. These patients often require modifying inserts, shoe modifications, or custom foot orthoses. The goal of these orthotic options is to distribute pressure forces evenly, help heal existing wounds, prevent new wounds, restore structural stability, and facilitate an energy-efficient gait.

Off-loading Orthotics and Prosthetics

A variety of shoe options are available for off-loading, especially in plantar-apexed deformities, such as Charcot neuroarthropathy, and in deformities associated with trauma, neuromuscular disorders, and congenital defects. Surgical shoes can be rocker bottom or flat in nature. For specific off-loading of lesions, removable hexagonal cutouts are available. For off-loading of the forefoot and rear foot, Darco orthowedge and heelwedge orthotics are available options. These shoes can make ambulation difficult; thus, supervised gait training with an assist device should be considered in these patients.

Extra-depth shoes provide an increased toe box height to accommodate deformities, such as rigid hammertoe contractures. The depth is increased by at least a quarter inch.

Custom diabetic shoes allow for accommodation using flexible material to allow for rigid hammertoe contractures and distal bony prominences. They typically have an accommodative insert that may be combined with custom posting or modification for biomechanical off-loading.

Rocker-bottom shoes off-load plantar pressure in the forefoot. The rocker addition allows for transition from heel strike to toe push-off. The biomechanical effects of the rocker soles aid in lost motion at the ankle joint. This modification also can progress the center of pressure beyond partial foot amputations and work to off-load areas of high pressure in the forefoot.

Orthotics

The distribution of peak pressures of the plantar foot is vital for healing chronic wounds, especially in neuropathic patients. Pressure mapping provides a good representation of concentrated pressure points on the plantar foot before orthotic use and shows the improved distribution of plantar pressures when the orthotic is worn (**Fig. 3**). Custom fit orthotics are valuable in the management of pressure-inducing deformities secondary to Charcot neuroarthropathy, trauma, neuromuscular disorders, and congenital defects. Custom fit orthoses may be used preoperatively, but after surgical intervention, they usually need to be modified to accommodate peak plantar pressures. Custom fit orthoses should be utilized for all patients suffering from wounds and diabetic peripheral neuropathy with or without pressure points. Pressure mapping clearly demonstrates the dispersion of peak forces that facilitates wound prevention

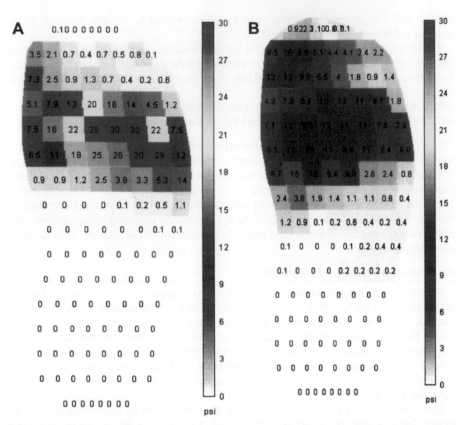

Fig. 3. (*A*) Pressure mapping obtained before soft inserts prescribed. Note the increased forefoot pressures that place chronic wounds at risk for nonhealing prior to soft inserts. (*B*) Pressure mapping obtained after soft inserts. Note the improved distribution of plantar pressures. (Copyright 2020, Dr. Christopher Bibbo, FACS/Main Street Enterprises-Globus Medical, LLC.)

as well as pressure relief during wound treatment (**Fig. 4**). An alternative to provide relief for a single wound is to mark the lesion with a marker prior to any foot casting or other technique used to construct a soft wound-unloading orthosis. A cutout then can be paired to the marked lesion.

After amputation, custom orthoses can be used perioperatively for protection of a new foot structure (eg, soft durometer shoe filler). In neuropathic patients where off-loading is desired for chronic wounds, one of the most common orthotic top layers for pressure relief is a light-weight polyethylene foam, cross-linked for durability (see **Fig. 4**). Ethylene-vinyl acetate also may be used to construct a soft custom orthosis (**Fig. 5**). An elastomeric polymer, ethylene-vinyl acetate demonstrates restoration of the physical state after compression, similar to flip-flops. In the construction of soft orthotics, multiple layers often are preferred. When wounds require significant local off-loading, upper layers may be stacked and a cutout provided. In the cutout, a silicone well may be made by placing silicone gel into the cutout. It must be stressed that all custom inserts that assist in the management of wounds must extend the full length of the existing foot. This ensures proper off-loading and distribution of ground-reactive forces not only for the wound but also for all other

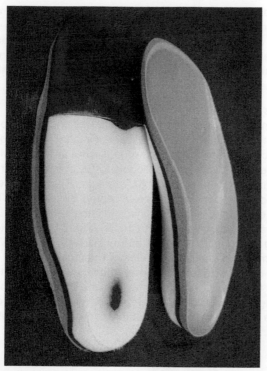

Fig. 4. This triple-layer soft insert is designed to accommodate a heel pressure point. (Copyright 2020, Dr. Christopher Bibbo, FACS/Main Street Enterprises-Globus Medical, LLC.)

pressure points. If a more functional insert is desired after wounds are healed and all pressure points resolved, the orthosis may be created using a base layer of higher density, such as cork/leather, with an upper layer of very conforming antishear materials. Different modalities for casting/molding custom orthotics are available for providers. Techniques can be use, such as plaster casting, direct to the skin, with simulated weight bearing and the ankle and subtalar joint in neutral. Other methods include pressure scanning, where weight bearing should be simulated while scanning a patient's feet. The simulated weight bearing should be performed with the ankle and subtalar joint in neutral.

Orthotic modifications aim at increasing or decreasing motion in certain areas of the foot. In cases of hallux limitus with chronic ulceration of the hallux tip, modifications

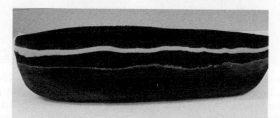

Fig. 5. A soft synthetic multilayer insert may provide stability with raising of the edges as well as distribution of forces. (Copyright 2020, Dr. Christopher Bibbo, FACS/Main Street Enterprises-Globus Medical, LLC.)

are made to increase the first metatarsophalangeal joint and decrease subsequent dispersion pressure. These modifications include a reverse Morton extension and first ray cutout. When discussing hallux rigidus, a Morton extension modification may be useful. This decreases the excursion at the first metatarsophalangeal joint, altering plantar loading patterns. Silicone heel lifts are another orthotic modification to reduce pressure off the heel.

Off-loading boots

Removable walking boots with controlled ankle motion (CAM) boots that possess removable padding to accommodate pressure points are helpful to off-load wounds during healing or can be used for healed wounds while being transitioned to a permanent device. Off-loading boots are applicable to Charcot neuroarthropathy, trauma, neuromuscular disorders, and congenital defects. These devices are less time consuming to apply and generally more accepted by patients. These CAM boots may be removed easily to facilitate local wound care.

The Charcot restraint orthotic walker (CROW) (**Fig. 6**A) is a custom-molded, rigid device containing appropriate areas of soft unloading. The CROW is preferred for high-grade deformities, particularly for Charcot neuroarthropathy. Charcot patients and patients with other conditions, however, must have a foot contour that is braceable. This implies that major bone prominences and severe deformities that interfere with brace making must be corrected. Typically, the CROW is a clamshell style to disperse pressure up the leg when an unstable midfoot, rear foot, or ankle is present.

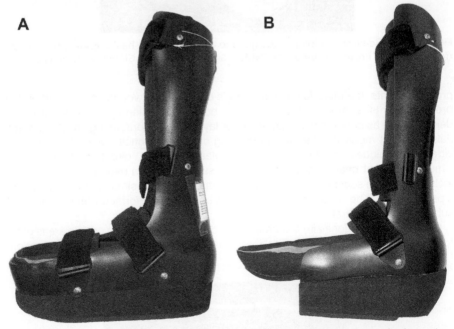

A

B

Fig. 6. (*A*) The standard CROW is a custom-molded brace designed to keep the lower leg, foot, and ankle snugly constrained. It is a workhorse brace in Charcot patients who are poor candidates for surgery. A thick soft insert is used for pressure point accommodation. Note the plantar external lift to accommodate for a limb length discrepancy. (*B*) Modified CROW boot for forefoot unloading. An anterior clam shell is important to prevent anterior translation of the tibia and shearing in the sagittal plane. (Copyright 2020, Dr. Christopher Bibbo, FACS/Main Street Enterprises-Globus Medical, LLC.)

A CROW is made of an outer polypropylene shell and inner layers of pressure relief inserts. Modifications of the CROW can be designed to off-load the forefoot, less commonly the heel (**Fig. 6**B).

Custom bracing
Biomechanical dysfunction of the ankle may contribute to the formation of any foot or ankle wound. The AFO is an indispensable brace for off-loading of multiple types of pressure wounds of the forefoot, midfoot, rearfoot, and ankle region. The AFO is most applicable to Charcot neuroarthropathy, but patients with trauma, neuromuscular disorders, and congenital defects also may benefit. Typically, an AFO is indicated when wounds in part hinge on the ankle function. Thus, the orthosis off-loads a fixed or motion segment. All AFOs must have several features: a soft, accommodating pressure-relief liner throughout the device, thicker relief inserts over the sole, and a silicone well, as needed. Vent holes drilled in the calf section help wick away excessive moisture. The AFO is designed to provide pressure relief by sharing the distribution of ground-reactive forces to more proximal regions, bypassing pathologic influences of the ankle complex. The AFO's terminating forces exit over the calf (standard AFO), the femoral condyles (femoral condyle–bearing AFO), and the patellar tendon (patellar-bearing AFO).

Two basic AFO ankle constructs are available:

- Solid AFOs: nonarticulating AFOs used when motion must be restricted. They usually are prescribed for support of unstable joints.
- Articulating AFOs: these are used when ankle motion is desired in effort to improve gait.

Features then are added to these 2 types of AFOs for specific needs. When a calcaneus gait causes loss of function of the gastrocnemius-soleus complex and severe pressure localized to the plantar calcaneus, it may result in one of the most difficult wounds to heal: the plantar calcaneal wound. To mitigate excessive plantar heel pressures, either a solid or an articulating dorsiflexion-stop AFO is implemented (**Fig. 7**). When calcaneal height has been lost after reconstruction (eg, partial calcanectomy with PMA flap), an internal silicone heel lift is placed. The appropriate height of the silicone heel is determined on plain radiographs by the complete covering of a native ankle or a relatively normal relationship between the first metatarsal/midfoot/talus (angulation between bones is relatively straight). A plantarflexion-stop AFO is placed for simple plantar heel protection for at-risk skin when ankle motion is desired and an abnormal fixed or dynamic plantarflexion is present (equinus deformity). When anterior compartment weakness is present, a dorsiflexion-assist AFO may be used.

A specific forefoot healing AFO may be constructed, consisting of a leg-restraining clamshell section, a custom-molded semiconstrained foot plate, and a custom pressure-relief soft liner. The extra height sole then may be reduced to produce a hybrid AFO/CROW boot.

The double upright calf lacer (DUCL) brace (**Fig. 8**) historically has been used in motor paralysis, such as poliomyelitis. The DUCL brace provides several biomechanical features, however, that are desirable to help treat wounds about the ankle all the while controlling ankle and rearfoot instability. The DUCL brace eliminates direct contact between the brace and the foot, and the ground-reactive forces are transmitted directly to the proximal leg and lower knee. The DUCL struts are clipped into a lined, rocker-bottom shoe and travel up the leg attaching to a proximal circular recipient for the uprights. The uprights often are stainless steel and may have a swing phase hinge that locks in the foot-flat phase of gait, providing significant ankle unloading. The DUCL,

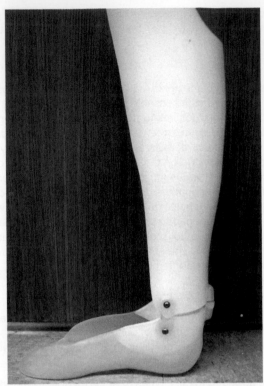

Fig. 7. The AFO is designed to control the ankle and rearfoot. The articulating hinge allows ankle motion, but the posterior stop design prevents excess plantar flexion, which is helpful in gastrocnemius-soleus weakness that imparts a calcaneus gait and plantar heel wounds, which are some of the most difficult to heal. (Copyright 2020, Dr. Christopher Bibbo, FACS/Main Street Enterprises-Globus Medical, LLC.)

however, imparts significant changes in the gait cycle, often restricting the use of the DUCL.

For completeness, the hinged knee AFO (KAFO) (**Fig. 9**) provides off-loading above the knee to the thigh and is useful especially with concomitant knee pathology. Motion may be allowed or locked through both the ankle and knee. All specifications of the standard AFO may be incorporated into the KAFO. Even more proximal designs provide off-loading to the level of the hip. These off-loading braces should be used for a narrow range of conditions where foot/ankle/leg/knee/hip off-loading is necessary. These braces have a significant impediment on the normal gait cycle.

The Arizona brace (**Fig. 10**) originally was designed for the nonoperative management of a nonfunctional posterior tibial tendon. Loss of the posterior tibial tendon results in a severe flatfoot that may portend exposure of the talar head, bearing focal pressure on the plantar medial arch, ultimately resulting in an ulcer (**Fig. 11**). When the talonavicular joint is still able to be manually reduced, the Arizona brace provides significant off-loading. From a functional standpoint, the Arizona brace is a gauntlet that acts like a miniature version of an AFO. The restriction of ankle motion, however, is less powerful, allowing better ankle function during gait. Typically, the Arizona brace is constructed of molded plastic that extends to the midlength of the foot, with an

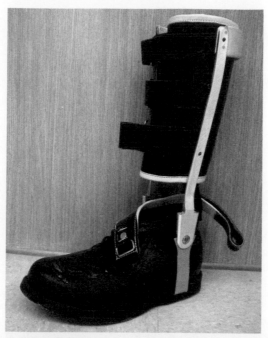

Fig. 8. DUCL brace provides significant off-loading through the ankle while allowing ankle range of motion. A rocker-bottom shoe is accommodative for pressure relieving inserts and the transitions through the phases of gate, allowing rapid transition from stance phase to toe-off in the gate cycle. (Copyright 2020, Dr. Christopher Bibbo, FACS/Main Street Enterprises-Globus Medical, LLC.)

interior-exterior overlay of finely padded leather that possesses lace eyelets or hook-and-loop fasteners.

For all patients, especially in patients with at-risk skin, existing wounds or postoperative status, the authors adhere to a strict prescription of the device being casted non–weight bearing with the joints placed in the neutral position and the use of a full-length footplate with a soft liner. In foot amputees, as for all amputee orthotics, the full-length footplate is finished with a soft durometer shoe filler. If needed, a high arch support, silicone well, or silicone heel pad is incorporated.

Total contact casting

Total contact casts (TCCs) were the first technique to provide ulcer off-loading. For decades, the TCC was considered the gold standard for off-loading the deformed foot with chronic plantar wounds, and it still has a role in managing chronic wounds. This device works by off-loading the foot while allowing the patient to ambulate. Ulcerations or high areas of pressure are protected, distributing pressure evenly throughout the adjacent region. As originally described, a plaster cast was applied directly over the skin so that the cast completely contacted the limb and allowed limited motion and equal weight distribution. Subsequently, the use of a minimum of padding was introduced before applying the cast, with the thought that tender skin was better protected. Over time, more padding was used to create a level weight-bearing surface that distributes pressure evenly or allows for pressure relief at critical areas. Minimal padding is used to allow the cast to completely contact the limb, allowing for limited motion and equal weight distribution. The TCC may be constructed of plaster,

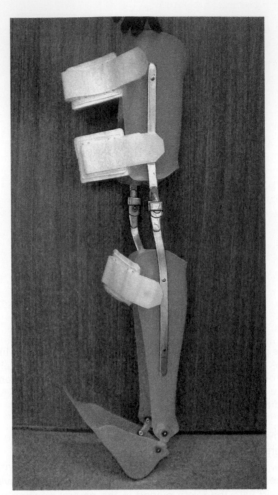

Fig. 9. Hinged KAFO relieves pressure by off-loading through the knee and ankle. KAFO may have a variety of joint designs. In this instance, the knee and ankle articulate. The ankle has a spring-loaded hinge that promotes ankle dorsiflexion, which is helpful when anterior compartment function is compromised. (Copyright 2020, Dr. Christopher Bibbo, FACS/Main Street Enterprises-Globus Medical, LLC.)

fiberglass, or a combination of a plaster underlayer that provides good foot contour and a fiberglass outer layer that provides strength.

As with any device, there also exists a downside of the TCC. The main concern of TTC is recidivism of the chronic wound as well as the occurrence of new ulcers. Although healing has been reported in 90% of patients after 5 weeks of TTC application, there was a 31% rate of wound recurrence and new ulcer formations.[14] The authors have found that the use of a self-adhering glycerine-based gel/hydrophilic polymer sheet (Elasto-Gel wound dressings, Southwest Technologies, North Kansas City, Missouri) in combination with a TCC (Jensen-style TCC), significantly mitigates recurrence of ulcers and the formation of new ulcerations. This occurs not only by padding the area but also by reducing wound edema and the bacteriostatic action of glycerin.[15]

The concerns of recurrent ulceration and new ulcer formation, dictate that the TCC be changed weekly. The TCC is best applied by an experienced clinician or cast

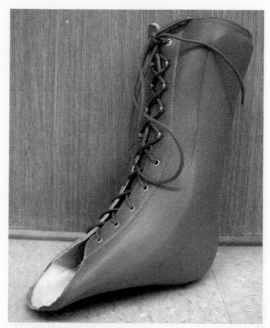

Fig. 10. A custom molded leather-metal ankle gauntlet can provide stability for mild flatfoot, allowing off-loading of medial foot chronic wounds around the arch. (Copyright 2020, Dr. Christopher Bibbo, FACS/Main Street Enterprises-Globus Medical, LLC.)

technician familiar with the TCC. Recently, a proprietary prepackaged TCC (Cutimed Off-Loader Select, BSN Medical, Hamburg, Germany) has been introduced. The proprietary TCC product reduces the time required to apply a TCC and thus has been met with great success. Once wounds are healed, custom inserts and shoes are made. During the transition from TCC to custom inserts/shoes, off-loading platform shoes or pressure-relief walking CAM boots are used.

OPERATIVE OFF-LOADING
External Fixation for Immediate Ambulation After Soft Tissue Reconstruction of Chronic Wounds

The most common method of patient mobilization after surgical reconstruction of chronic foot and ankle wounds has been to require patients to be non–weight bearing with crutches, walkers, or a wheelchair. The recent use of knee scooters has helped young, healthy patients, who are a minority in the chronic wound population. Often patients are older, have more complex medical comorbidities, and are deconditioned. These patients cannot comply with the prescribed weight-bearing status with these methods, which leads to deconditioning, depression, and noncompliance. Noncompliance quickly leads to failure of the reconstructive effort. Limited mobility also may lead to social isolation, which may worsen these postoperative complications. Thus, these most common methods of mobilization and protection of the operative site put reconstructive techniques (eg, flaps and skin grafts) in significant jeopardy. These issues result in longer hospital and rehabilitation facility lengths of stay, with an increase in expenditures of health care costs.

The use of external fixation to protect soft tissue reconstruction of wounds, such as flaps and skin grafts, was first described in 2007 to off-load a PMA flap to cover a

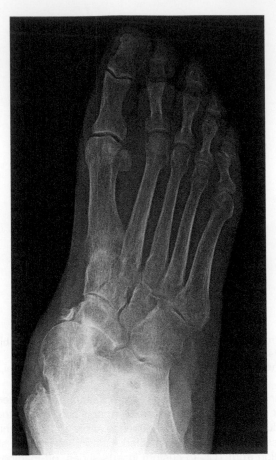

Fig. 11. Anteroposterior-view radiograph of severe pes planus (flatfoot) with protrusion of the talar head. The subtalar joint axis induces motion in 3 planes; thus, the head lands plantar-medial rotated. This places the plantar medial foot at significant risk for developing a wound. Due to the focal and very high sustained force, acute wounds quickly become chronic without reconstruction followed by prosthetic off-loading. (Copyright 2020, Dr. Christopher Bibbo, FACS/Main Street Enterprises-Globus Medical, LLC.)

chronic heel wound with osteomyelitis (**Fig. 12**).(ref) Subsequently, the technique was refined with applicability to any plantar wound and other extremity wounds needing off-loading protection. This technique uses a circular external fixator, fine wires, and/or half-pins. These allow immediate progressive weight bearing while protecting the healing of wounds and the wound reconstructions. **Fig. 13** demonstrates the use of an external fixator to off-load a reverse sural flap from posterior and plantar pressures while also protecting the donor site and negative-pressure wound dressing. The patient is allowed full weight bearing with a walker on postoperative day 1 (see **Fig. 13**). Additionally, correction of abnormalities in bone architecture may be corrected at the same time with osteotomies, fusions, and distraction osteogenesis. The use of external fixation for soft tissue protection with immediate ambulation has proved beneficial for the orthoplastic management of lower extremity wounds throughout the entire perioperative period (this technique may be used in the upper extremity).

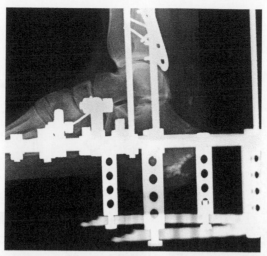

Fig. 12. Lateral-view radiograph of a posterior heel wound being off-loaded for ambulation prior to surgery, which then will allow ambulation after a flap. (Copyright 2020, Dr. Christopher Bibbo, FACS/Main Street Enterprises-Globus Medical, LLC.)

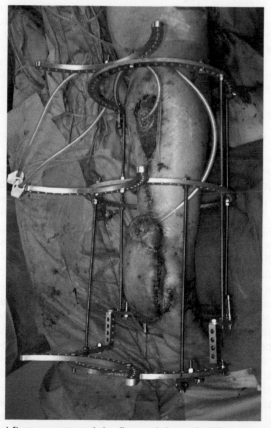

Fig. 13. The external fixator protected the flap and donor bed from external pressure while allowing immediate weight bearing. (Copyright 2020, Dr. Christopher Bibbo, FACS/Main Street Enterprises-Globus Medical, LLC.)

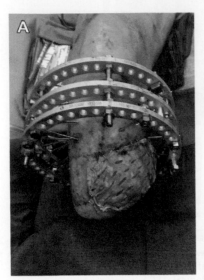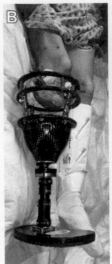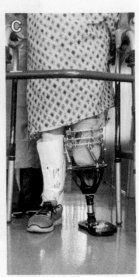

Fig. 14. (*A*) Clinical photograph of a below-knee amputation with skin graft over a muscle flap to preserve the level of the amputation. This is an example where an external fixation–based postoperative prosthesis provides access to continued wound care and protects the soft tissue reconstruction. (*B*) The X-Prosthesis IPOP allows immediate, full weight-bearing ambulation on postoperative day 1. It also protects surgical incisions and allows monitoring and continued care of stump reconstructions. (*C*) Patient ambulating using the X-Prosthesis IPOP and a walker. Note complete off-loading and access to amputation site. When healing is complete, the prosthesis allows unrestricted showering. (Copyright 2020, Dr. Christopher Bibbo, FACS/Main Street Enterprises-Globus Medical, LLC)

External Fixation–Based Prosthetic Device for Immediate Ambulation After Major Amputations

Based on the success of external fixation techniques to protect foot and ankle wound reconstruction, an external fixator–based immediate postoperative prosthesis (IPOP) for major lower extremity amputations has been developed (X-Prosthesis, Postop Innovations, Fallston, Maryland). Conventional IPOPs have demonstrated significant limitations, requiring a near-normal skin condition, a more robust patient, and only partial weight bearing. Even in contemporary reports, conventional IPOPs do not allow for inspection of the skin of the amputated limb, much less the incision.[16]

In contrast, the X-Prosthesis IPOP (**Fig. 14**) allows immediate, full weight-bearing ambulation on postoperative day 1, while protecting surgical incisions and allowing monitoring and continued care of stump reconstructions (eg, local wound care, negative pressure dressings, skin grafts, and flaps). This early, full weight-bearing bipedal ambulation reduces deconditioning and has improved patient hospital depression scores, length of stay, participation in level 1 rehabilitation, and time to not only a temporary prosthesis but also permanent prosthesis. The X-Prosthesis has been used successfully in bilateral below-knee amputations as well as above-knee amputations. Below-knee amputations with knee flexion contractures are particularly difficult to manage, but they have been successfully managed with the X-Prosthesis by utilizing a gradual flexion deformity correction technique, while continuing with full weight-bearing ambulation starting on postoperative day 1.

SUMMARY

Foot and ankle deformities contribute to the genesis and perpetuation of chronic wounds. When deformity is present, bone and soft tissue pathology must be addressed either surgically or by nonoperative biomechanical control. Off-loading of soft tissue and bone via inserts, braces, and external fixation is pivotal in the multidisciplinary approach to the management of chronic wounds.

DISCLOSURE

The authors have nothing to disclose.

REFERENCES

1. Jäger M, Zilkens C, Zanger K, et al. Significance of nano- and microtopography for cell-surface interactions in orthopaedic implants. J Biomed Biotechnol 2007; 2007(8):69036.
2. Conlon BP, Nakayasu ES, Fleck LE, et al. Activated ClpP kills persisters and eradicates a chronic biofilm infection. Nature 2013;503(7476):365–70.
3. Reilly SS, Hudson MC, Kellam JF, et al. In vivo internalization of Staphylococcus aureus by embryonic chick osteoblasts. Bone 2000;26(1):63–70.
4. Hudson MC, Ramp WK, Nicholson NC, et al. Internalization of Staphylococcus aureus by cultured osteoblasts. Microb Pathog 1995;19(6):409–19.
5. Tucker KA, Reilly SS, Leslie CS, et al. Intracellular Staphylococcus aureus induces apoptosis in mouse osteoblasts. FEMS Microbiol Lett 2000;186(2):151–6.
6. Ellington JK, Harris M, Hudson MC, et al. Intracellular Staphylococcus aureus and antibiotic resistance: implications for treatment of staphylococcal osteomyelitis. J Orthop Res 2006;24(1):87–93.
7. Meagher J, Zellweger R, Filgueira L. Functional dissociation of the basolateral transcytotic compartment from the apical phago-lysosomal compartment in human osteoclasts. J Histochem Cytochem 2005;53(5):665–70.
8. Miller MB, Bassler BL. Quorum sensing in bacteria. Annu Rev Microbiol 2001;55: 165–99.
9. Konaklieva MI, Plotkin BJ. Chemical communication–do we have a quorum? Mini Rev Med Chem 2006;6(7):817–25.
10. Bibbo C. Modification of the Syme amputation to prevent postoperative heel pad migration. J Foot Ankle Surg 2013;52(6):766–70.
11. Greene CJ, Bibbo C. The lisfranc amputation: a more reliable level of amputation with proper intraoperative tendon balancing. J Foot Ankle Surg 2017;56(4):824–6.
12. Bibbo C, Stough JD. Reduction calcaneoplasty and local muscle rotation flap as a salvage option for calcaneal osteomyelitis with soft tissue defect. J Foot Ankle Surg 2012;51(3):375–8.
13. Bibbo C. External fixator assisted immediate wound closure. Tech Foot Ankle Surg 2006;5(3):144–9.
14. Myerson M, Papa J, Eaton K, et al. The total-contact cast for management of neuropathic plantar ulceration of the foot. J Bone Joint Surg Am 1992;74(2):261–9.
15. Stout EI, McKessor A. Glycerin-based hydrogel for infection control. Adv Wound Care (New Rochelle) 2012;1(1):48–51.
16. Ali MM, Loretz L, Shea A, et al. A contemporary comparative analysis of immediate postoperative prosthesis placement following below-knee amputation. Ann Vasc Surg 2013;27(8):1146–53.

Biofilm and Chronic Nonhealing Wound Infections

Steven R. Evelhoch, MD, DDS, FACS, MMHC, MBA

KEYWORDS

- Biofilm infections • Biofilm • Nonhealing wound

KEY POINTS

- Many chronic nonhealing wound infections are caused by biofilm formation.
- Diagnosing biofilm infections can be difficult because of their nature of adherence and multilayering.
- Biofilm infections are associated with implantable medical devices and host tissue.
- Treatment of biofilm infections is difficult with current means and will require new technology, new antimicrobials, and new therapies.

INTRODUCTION

Patients with chronic nonhealing wounds represent approximately 15% of Medicare beneficiaries.[1] Total Medicare spending estimates are close to $100 billion.[1] Surgical infections are the largest source of chronic infections, followed by diabetic infections.[1] Chronic nonhealing wounds include venous leg ulcers, diabetic foot ulcers, pressure ulcers, and burns. Biofilms are found in most chronic infections and especially on implanted medical devices, such as artificial heart valves.[2,3]

PATHOGENESIS

Bacteria are the oldest life forms on Earth.[2] Bacteria have developed capabilities to survive and thrive. One of these capabilities is to colonize and form biofilms.[2] Biofilm is a thick layer of prokaryotic organisms that have aggregated to form a colony.[2] The colony attaches to a surface with a polysaccharide layer called the slime layer.[2] The slime layer is also known as the extracellular polymeric substance or EPS.[2] The EPS consists of polysaccharides, extracellular DNA, proteins, lipids, biosurfactants, flagella, and pili.[2] The EPS protects the microorganisms by forming around and over the growing colony.[2] This biofilm promotes growth of the colony and protects it from threats to survival.[2] The biofilm is porous to allow for nutrients and elimination

No financial interest in any company.
Department of Oral and Maxillofacial Surgery, Marshfield Medical Center, 1000 North Oak Avenue, Marshfield, WI 54449, USA
E-mail address: evelhoch.steven@marshfieldclinic.org

Surg Clin N Am 100 (2020) 727–732
https://doi.org/10.1016/j.suc.2020.05.004

of waste products.[2] Bacterial growth is characterized by 2 phenotypes: single cells called planktonic and sessile aggregates.[2] The planktonic bacteria are free-floating single cells.[2] The first observation of sessile aggregates was made by observing dental plaque.[2] The biofilm can be composed of gram-positive bacteria, gram-negative bacteria, or a combination of both.[2]

The biofilm is formed when even 1 cell attaches to a surface. The first cells produce proteins that signal other nearby cells. These signals recruit other cells into the new colony. As the number of cells grows, biofilm is then produced by the production of polysaccharides, which is the beginning of the EPS. In most biofilms, the microorganisms account for less than 10% of the dry mass. The matrix can account for more than 90%.

The colony is protected by the biofilm, which grows along with the biofilm. This arrangement is a cooperative arrangement that brings nutrients into the colony and allows for the survival of the colony. The microorganisms share genetic material, which also enhances the survival of the colony. The biofilm protects the microorganisms from flow of fluids, the host's immune system, and antibiotics.[2]

Biofilm Theory

Pseudomonas aeruginosa infections in patients with cystic fibrosis were reported as early as 1977. These infections were described as clumps or heaps of bacteria. Dr John William Costerton from the University of Copenhagen pioneered the development of the biofilm theory. In 1978, he described a glycocalyx matrix and in 1981 was the first to coin the term biofilm. Today the Costerton Biofilm Center in Copenhagen is a leading center for biofilm research. In 1999, Costerton defined biofilm as a "structured community of bacterial cells enclosed in a self-produced polymeric matrix adherent to a surface."[2]

Studies have shown that acute infections are often the result of planktonic forms of bacteria, yeast, and parasites. These microorganisms float freely throughout the body. These are treated by antibiotics and antimicrobial medications. Once the organisms have formed a biofilm, the infection often proceeds to a chronic status and is resistant to antibiotics, antimicrobials, and the host's immune system.[2]

Chronic Infections

Biofilms are found in irritable bowel syndrome, tympanic membranes, chronic wound infections, osteomyelitis, dental plaque, pseudomonal lung infections in cystic fibrosis patients, tonsillitis, implants, artificial heart valves, contact lenses, and all types of indwelling catheters.[2] Biofilm antibiotic tolerance is different from biofilm antibiotic resistance. Bacteria embedded in a biofilm are able to survive antibiotic and antimicrobial treatment in both tolerance and resistance, but when the biofilm is disrupted, the bacteria now are susceptible to antibiotic treatment. Acute infections usually involve the planktonic forms of microorganisms, including parasites, yeast, and bacteria.[2] Once the biofilm is produced, the infection often becomes chronic and resistant to antimicrobial agents and the host immune system.[2] The bacteria in the biofilm are physically joined and produce an extracellular matrix. Microorganisms in the biofilm can communicate with 1 another via signaling known as quorum sensing.[2] Infection is a common problem with chronic wounds. There is an increased risk of patient morbidity and mortality. Delayed healing, pain, compromise of the immune response, resistance to antibiotics, nosocomial infections, and the increased cost to society are substantial.[2] There is an increase in intensive care unit stay and operating room visits.[1,2] Several factors contribute to the transition from colonization to infection, including virulence of the microorganisms, susceptibility of the host, the bioburden of the microorganisms, and the sharing of the genetic material between the microorganisms.[2]

Wounds provide the ideal environment for the development of biofilm. The extracellular matrix components, such as collagen, fibronectin, and laminin, serve as attachment components for the microorganisms.[2] Wound beds are moist, have the proper pH, and are nutritious allowing for development of the microcolonies.[4] Bacterial cultures are difficult to obtain from biofilm, and debridement alone does not effectively eradicate the biofilm.[4] Some studies estimate 60% of chronic infections is due to biofilm formation.[2] It is more difficult to culture and obtain Gram stains on bacteria residing in a biofilm.[2] A chronic infection can display normal flora because of the biofilm. Debridement of a bacterial biofilm can be ineffective because of bacteria being driven deep into tissues. Often a recurrence of infection will occur.[4]

Staphylococcus aureus bacteria cause numerous chronic infections and are at the root of the problems in community-acquired and nosocomial infections.[5] With its ability to form a biofilm, the understanding of its impact on chronic wounds continues to grow.[5] Because of biofilm-associated drug resistance, the treatment of chronic wounds can be arduous (**Table 1**).[5]

Diagnosis

The diagnosis of biofilm infection is primarily by clinical findings. Biofilm resistance is multifactorial and may vary greatly from 1 infection to another. Bacteria within a biofilm can resist up to a 1000-fold concentration of antibiotics even if the same bacteria are susceptible in the planktonic state. Various mechanisms are thought to be responsible for antibiotic resistance. Hypotheses include antibiotic resistance to penetration of the biofilm, the microenvironment of the biofilm itself with the very deep layers of the biofilm being hypoxic, or by phenotypical differentiation.

The most commonly studied bacterium is *P aeruginosa*. *P aeruginosa* is a gram-negative, nonfermentative organism facultative anaerobe. The ability of this bacterium to form a biofilm is one of its main survival strategies. Most of the biofilm produced by *P aeruginosa* consists of water channels; these are thought to function for distributing

Table 1 Biofilm-associated infections	
Medical Devices Associated with Infections	**Tissue Associated with Infections**
Breast implants	Breast tissue
Cardiovascular implantable devices	Biliary tract
Catheters, shunts, and stents	Internal ear
Cochlear implants	Tonsils
Contact lenses	Sinuses
Deep brain stimulators	Wounds
Endotracheal tubes	Teeth
Vascular grafts	Blood vessels
Fixation plates and screws	Kidney stones
	Lung (cystic fibrosis)
	Bone (osteomyelitis)

Data from Hoiby N, Bjarnsholt T, Moser C, et al. ESCMID guideline for the diagnosis and treatment of biofilm infections 2014. Clin Microbiol Infect 2015;21 Suppl 1:S1–25.

nutrients and oxygen. Nutrient availability is one of the most important factors affecting colonization. The oxygen gradient descends from the biofilm's surface to its substratum.[2]

Biofilm Development

The biofilm developmental process can be divided into 4 stages: attachment, microcolony formation, maturation, and dispersion. The biofilm is thought to maintain equilibrium by growth and then by dispersion. Dispersion can occur by release of single cells or microcolonies.[2] Dispersion provides a mechanism whereby bacteria can spread throughout the body from a chronic infection causing an acute infection at a different location, as can be seen with infected artificial heart valves caused by infected teeth.[2]

Treatment

There are 4 main strategies in treating biofilm infections.[6] The first strategy is to prevent initial contamination of a device by maintaining optimal aseptic technique and minimizing the duration of time that the device is in vivo.[6] The second strategy is to take steps to minimize initial microbial attachment by using an antibiotic-coated device.[6] Third is to use agents that can penetrate a biofilm, such as high doses of antibiotics along with future development of biofilm matrix disrupters.[6] The fourth strategy is removal of the infected device during definitive treatment.[6]

Detection

Because of the very nature of biofilms, detecting them is challenging. Several methods have been found to detect biofilms in a laboratory setting, but this has not translated to the clinical setting. Biofilm infections are generally associated with chronic infections. Biofilm infections also remain at local infection sites with implanted devices. Biofilms can produce occult or subclinical infections, which elicit a diminished host inflammatory response, and therefore, they are more difficult to detect and treat.

When a biofilm is formed on an implanted device, it cannot be detected without removal.[7] Even then, detection can be difficult with current microbiological methods, such as culturing in the laboratory. Even if cells are detected, slow-growing variants and persister cells may not form colonies in the laboratory setting.[7] Current culturing techniques can be ineffective because of the heterogeneity of biofilms and the involvement of mixed species biofilms and the involvement of fastidious strains of bacteria.[7] A standardized technique for detection of biofilms in a clinical setting has yet to be developed. This area is an area in which molecular techniques are showing promise.

Recent advances in biofilm detection include molecular methods, biofilm-associated biomarkers, and biofilm imaging. Molecular methods include metagenomic sequencing from DNA-based technologies.[7] Compared with polymerase chain reaction–based approaches that target ribosomal RNA for detection, metagenomic sequencing based on DNA technologies can reveal more information, such as antibiotic resistance and virulence factors.[7] The development of whole-genomic sequencing has improved throughput, accuracy, and cost of biofilm detection.[7] Biofilm-associated biomarkers can detect unique molecules or stimulate a biofilm-specific host response. Antibodies may not be detected during an acute infection but can be used to detect a biofilm-associated infection. An example of this is the detection of alpha defensin, an antimicrobial peptide produced by the body to fight infection, which has been found in the synovial fluid of infected hip and knee joints. Besides host factors, biofilm-specific markers on bacterial cells will enable detection of biofilms. A biofilm-associated protein (Bap) has been discovered in S aureus. Bap homologues have been discovered in other bacteria. Biofilm imaging provides methods for biofilm culturing, imaging, and analysis by providing spatial information about biofilms. Unconventional methods, such as bioimpedance-based sensing using electric currents and surface acoustic waves using vibration, are also promising in detection of biofilms.

New Therapies

Detection is only 1 component of biofilm treatment. New therapies are being developed to prevent and control biofilm-related infections. Surface coating or eluting substrates and other approaches for inhibiting initial bacterial attachment and recent advances in surface technologies and materials have shown promise.[7] One of the more intriguing treatments is phage therapy. Bacteriophages are natural predators of bacteria. Studies have shown that phages can infect and lyse cells present in single and polymicrobial species biofilms. The close proximity of cells in a biofilm could make the phages more effective in facilitating an infection. The biofilm structure could also be an obstacle to phage infection. Phage-biofilm interactions are highly dependent on the bacterial host strain, the phage characteristics, and biofilm structure and composition.[8,9]

The use of bacteriophages for biofilm prevention is promising, but many limitations exist. The biofilm matrix along with the reduced metabolic activity of biofilm cells and phage-resistant phenotypes are current barriers to eradication of the biofilm.[8] Phages need to reach their targets and attach to specific receptors located at the cell surface of bacteria.[8] Phage access to planktonic bacteria is easier than bacterial access in biofilms.[8]

Strategies to enhance biofilm control by phages include mechanical debridement, combination therapy using antibiotics and antiseptics, combined therapy with enzymes, phage cocktails, and genetic manipulation of phages.[8] Mechanical debridement causes disruption of the biofilm enhancing the phage infection because of better accessibility to the biofilm cells. Combination therapy with antibiotics and antiseptics has been shown to enhance biofilm eradication.[8] Using a phage infection before antibiotic use or antiseptic use has shown to control *P aeruginosa* biofilm growth.[8] Combined phage therapy with enzymes has shown to be promising as well.[8] Depolymerases are polysaccharide-degrading enzymes that have been studied and shown to degrade the biofilm.[8] Phage cocktails using multiple phages with different host ranges and targeting of different receptors are used in the biofilm.[8] Genetic manipulation includes the development of new phages designed for specific bacterial targets.[8]

SUMMARY

Biofilm infections consist of organized communities of microorganisms embedded within a matrix. The complete eradication of biofilms is one of the major hurdles to healing chronic wounds. These structures are complex and not completely understood. They are difficult to study in the clinical environment. They have developed survival techniques that change rapidly. They are resistant to single therapies. The host responses can vary with a biofilm infection. The continued development of new strategies is promising, but the challenges for treatment remain. Chronic nonhealing wounds with biofilm infections will continue to impact the health care system.

REFERENCES

1. Nussbaum SR, Carter MJ, Fife CE, et al. An economic evaluation of the impact, cost, and Medicare policy implications of chronic non-healing wounds. Value Health 2018;21:27–32.

2. Bjarnsholt T. The role of bacterial biofilms in chronic infections. APMIS 2013; 121(136):1–54.
3. Wi YM, Patel R. Understanding biofilms and novel approaches to the diagnosis, prevention, and treatment of medical device-associated infections. Infect Dis Clin North Am 2018;32(4):915–29.
4. Sen C, Roy S, Gordillo G. Principles. 4th edition. Wound healing. Plastic surgery, vol. 1. St Louis (MO): Elsevier; 2018. p. 165–95.
5. Demir C, Demirci M, Yigin A, et al. Presence of biofilm and adhesin genes in Staphylococcus aureus strains taken from chronic wound infections and their genotypic and phenotypic antimicrobial sensitivity patterns. Photodiagnosis Photodyn Ther 2020;29(101584):1–5.
6. Aslam S. Effect of antibacterials on biofilms. Am J Infect Control 2008;36(10): S175.e9-11.
7. Xu Y, Dhaouadi Y, Stoodley P, et al. Understanding biofilms and novel approaches to the diagnosis, prevention, and treatment of medical device-associated infections. Curr Opin Biotechnol 2020;64:79–84.
8. Pires D, Melo L, Boas D, et al. Phage therapy as an alternative or complementary strategy to prevent and control biofilm-related infections. Curr Opin Microbiol 2017;39:48–56.
9. Garcia NM, Cai J. Aggressive soft tissue infections. Surg Clin North Am 2018; 98(5):1097–108.

Plastic Surgery Techniques for Wound Coverage

Brad T. Morrow, MD

KEYWORDS

- Wound reconstruction • Local flaps • Z-plasty • Surgical delay

KEY POINTS

- The most important concepts in flap-based wound reconstruction are designing a flap with an adequate blood supply.
- It is also important to ensure the flap is large enough to cover the intended wound and avoiding unnecessary tension on wound closure.
- Axial flaps incorporate a named vessel within the flap, whereas random flaps require careful planning because the flap is based on the subdermal vascular plexus for its blood supply.
- Surgical delay of a flap can be beneficial to improve the distal perfusion of a flap by allowing "choke" vessels to dilate and increase blood flow.

INTRODUCTION

The reconstruction of wounds has been a long recognized problem. The earliest documented techniques of wound reconstruction date back to 600 BC India when Sushruta Samita described a cheek flap for nasal wound coverage.[1,2] A crude understanding of wound coverage persisted into the sixteenth century when Gaspare Tagliacozzi refined a technique using a flap of arm skin to reconstruct nasal wounds. The word flap is derived from "flappe," a sixteenth-century Dutch term referring to an object that is attached by 1 side and hung loosely.[3] The modern concepts of wound coverage originated during World War II as an increasing number of soldiers survived their battlefield trauma and required extensive reconstruction with local or regional cutaneous and musculocutaneous flaps. Further refinements were elucidated as surgeons developed a more comprehensive understanding of the vascular anatomy of the human body. The advent of microsurgical techniques expanded the possibilities of wound coverage because tissue could be harvested from any part of the body. The evolution of techniques now defines a flap as a single or combination of tissue types (skin, muscle, fascia, or bone) that maintains its intrinsic blood supply when transferred from a donor to a recipient site.

Department of Plastic and Craniomaxillofacial Surgery, Marshfield Clinic Health System, 1000 North Oak Avenue, Mail Code 3F3, Marshfield, WI 54449, USA
E-mail address: morrow.brad@marshfieldclinic.org

Surg Clin N Am 100 (2020) 733–740
https://doi.org/10.1016/j.suc.2020.05.005
0039-6109/20/© 2020 Elsevier Inc. All rights reserved.

ANATOMY

The relevant anatomy of flaps is based on the vascular system. Designing a flap without an understanding of the vascular supply will be destined to fail.

Skin, consisting of the epidermis, papillary dermis, and reticular dermis, is primarily perfused via the subdermal vascular plexus, which traverses parallel between the reticular dermis and subcutaneous tissue (**Fig. 1**). This extensive plexus has numerous collateral connections and is supplied by septocutaneous or musculocutaneous perforating vessels, which travel through the fascial septae between muscles or directly through muscles respectively and are derived from named axial arteries.

The vascular system was exquisitely described when Taylor and Palmer[4] introduced the concept of an angiosome, which is a section of composite tissue (skin, subcutaneous tissue, muscle, and bone) that is perfused by a single source vessel and its perforating branches. Angiosomes are connected by choke vessels that can shunt blood between systems if the source is disrupted. Therefore, a flap designed on a single source vessel can perfuse neighboring territories during transfer. Understanding the angiosome system allows for the design of larger flaps that can be transferred in a safer and more reliable fashion.

FLAP CLASSIFICATION

The vascular system forms the basis for the classifications of flaps. Random flaps are not designed on a dominant vessel and are perfused via the subdermal plexus. Axial flaps incorporate a dominant named vessel, which allows for increased freedom in flap design. Axial flaps are further described by whether the source vessel is intact. A pedicled flap maintains an intact vessel, whereas a free flap ligates and divides the source vessel. Microsurgical techniques are required to anastomose the source donor vessel to a recipient vessel. A pedicled flap is limited by the reach of the source vessel, whereas a free flap's reach is limitless.

Flaps can also be described based on the included tissue types such as skin, fascia, muscle, or bone. A composite flap incorporates multiple tissue types into the design. The decision of which tissue types to include in a flap depends on the characteristics of the wound to be reconstructed. A shallow defect may be reconstructed with a flap consisting of skin, subcutaneous tissue, and superficial fascia. A deeper defect may

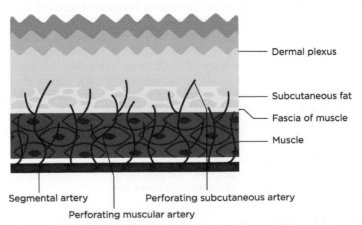

Fig. 1. The skin is perfused via the subdermal vascular plexus, which traverses parallel between the reticular dermis and subcutaneous tissue.

require additional bulk from a fasciocutaneous flap, which also includes the deep fascial system. A deep or contaminated defect may require the addition of muscle, which can obliterate dead space, improve the reach of the flap and has a robust vascular supply, which can help to eradicate bacterial contamination.[5] Musculocutaneous flaps have been classified based on their blood supply.[6] When planning to close a pressure ulcer, fasciocutaneous flaps are more resistant to pressure-induced ischemia as compared with muscle flaps, which are highly sensitive to ischemia. Wounds requiring structural support necessitate the addition of bone.

WOUND PREPARATION

Before definitive reconstruction, wounds must be critically evaluated and detrimental factors must be controlled. Chronic wounds necessitate a complete and thorough debridement to remove fibrinous debris and devitalized, necrotic, or infected tissue. The debridement is the most important step in wound coverage to prevent complications and improve chances for success. Chronic wound are generally contaminated with bacteria. The bacterial load should be kept below 10^5 bacteria per gram to enable wound healing and decrease the risk of flap loss.[7,8] Wounds should also be evaluated for ischemia, which may require adjunctive vascular intervention for healing.

Chronic wounds may be prepared for definitive reconstruction with the use of a vacuum-assisted closure device by removing exudate, edema, and other factors that can impair wound healing. It must be stated that a vacuum-assisted closure is not a substitute for an adequate debridement and should be avoided if devitalized tissue is still present.

TISSUE HANDLING

Proper tissue handling maintains respect for the tissue by avoiding unnecessary force or creating ischemic crush injuries to the skin. Excessive tension on the skin closure can compress the subdermal plexus and lead to flap necrosis or dehiscence.

RECONSTRUCTIVE LADDER (ELEVATOR)

The reconstructive ladder is a useful framework to approach wound coverage by assessing whether the simplest method would provide adequate treatment and then progressing in a stepwise fashion to more complex techniques. Wounds can be treated, from simplest to complex, by healing by secondary intention, primary closure, delayed primary closure, skin grafts, local flaps, regional flaps, and free tissue flaps. The main concept is selecting the least invasive technique that can reliably reconstruct the wound with the least morbidity. Each rung of the ladder does not have to be attempted and the concept has been expanded to an elevator framework, because simpler methods can be bypassed and more complex techniques can be selected initially if required to restore the form and function of the wound.

LOCAL FLAPS

Local flaps are generally chosen to reconstruct cutaneous defects that cannot be repaired in a straight line. Local flaps mobilize adjacent tissue and use the elasticity of the skin to close the defect. Wide undermining is performed to recruit tissue. The most important steps in designing a local flap is ensuring the vascular system can perfuse the flap and there is not significant tension on the closure. Insufficient blood flow or too much tension will lead to distal flap necrosis or wound dehiscence. Creating a flap slightly larger than anticipated may help to increase the blood supply and distance the flap can transfer. The state of the adjacent tissue must be assessed because inflamed and edematous tissue will never move as well as soft and supple tissue.

The viability of a flap may be increased by the delay phenomenon, in which a portion of the blood supply to a flap is divided without transferring the flap to reconstruct a defect. The relative ischemia created is not enough to cause tissue necrosis but instead can induce angiogenesis and vasodilatory factors that dilate "choke" vessels to increase blood flow from neighboring angiosomes.[9] The delay phenomenon typically requires 10 days to 2 weeks to achieve the maximum effect. Planning for delayed transfer of a flap may be prudent in the presence of an impaired microcirculation in smokers or diabetic patients. If transferring a flap results in ischemia or venous congestion, then returning the flap to its native position and allowing for the delay phenomenon to occur may be a reasonable alternative to avoid complications.

There are a wide variety of different types of local flaps and the decision of which type to use is based on characteristics of the wound and adjacent tissue.

Advancement Flaps

An advancement flap is the linear movement of tissue and is designed by making parallel incisions at the edge of a wound (**Fig. 2**). Undermining around the edge of a wound mobilizes tissue so that a smaller flap may be designed with less distance to advance and less tension on the closure. The flap should be elevated at a depth similar to the wound to improve the final aesthetic result. The flap may be tethered at the base or create standing cutaneous deformities or "dog ears" after the advancement. Excising triangles of tissue away from the base of the flap will release its movement and correct the dog ears. Care must be taken to avoid excising triangles of tissue toward the base of the flap because this technique will narrow the pedicle or base of the flap and may compromise the blood flow.

Single advancement flap

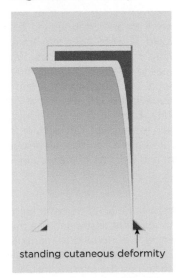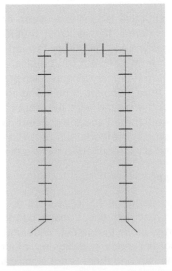

standing cutaneous deformity

Fig. 2. An advancement flap is the linear movement of tissue along parallel incisions at the edge of a wound.

An opposing advancement flap may also be designed to decrease the distance the flap must travel. This flap can be considered after the first flap is elevated and advanced to ensure that the second flap is adequate or necessary.

A variation of the advancement flap is the V-Y island pedicle flap, which is performed by making 2 incisions from the width of the defect that converge to an approximate 30° angle or V shape. The flap is described as an island because there is a complete circumferential incision around the flap and it is no longer perfused by the subdermal plexus but rather from perforating vessels arising from the deeper muscles or septum. The flap is elevated by undermining along the edges of the flap; care must be taken not to disturb the central deeper tissue, which is providing the blood supply. After the flap is advanced, the resulting suture line has the appearance of a Y.

Rotational Flaps

A rotational flap may be used if there is multidirectional skin laxity. A curved line is marked from the base of the defect to approximately one-third of a circle (**Fig. 3**). The flap is then rotated into the defect. The distal extent of the arc is the pivot point by which the flap will rotate. An excision of a triangle of tissue away from the base of the flap may further improve the rotation and eliminate a standing cutaneous deformity. A back cut into the base of the flap certainly improves the rotation but, again, it may jeopardize the blood supply to the flap.

Transposition Flaps

Transposition flaps use adjacent tissue, but are transposed over native tissue that remains in place. The main advantage of a transposition flap is that it can redistribute the vectors of tension on closure. There are 2 main types of a transposition flaps, the Z-plasty and rhomboid flap.

A Z-plasty is not used to close a defect, but instead to lengthen or rearrange tissue such as a contracted scar (**Fig. 4**). The design incorporates a central limb, which may be a scar or tissue to be lengthened, with 2 lateral limbs that are equal in length and the angle formed with the central limb. The lateral limbs should not extend past the midpoint of the central limb. The central limb is incised if tissue is to be lengthened or the scar is excised if it is causing a contracture. This technique forms 2 equal triangular flaps that, when transposed, will lengthen and reorient the central limb by 90°. The percentage by which the central limb is lengthened depends on the angles formed with the lateral limbs. Increasing the angle increases the length of the central limb. For example, a 30° angle increases the central limb by 25% whereas a 60° angle increases it by 75%. The 60° Z-plasty if most frequently used to maximize central limb length but minimize tension on the closure.

A rhomboid flap is marked by converting the defect into a parallelogram with equal lengths (x) and 60 and 120° angles (**Fig. 5**). A line of equal length (x) is marked from the 120° angle and forming another 120° angle. A second line of equal length (x) is marked from the distal extent staying parallel to the length of the defect and forming a 60° angle. After the flap is elevated and transposed, the vector of tension on the closure with be redirected by 90°.

Regional Flaps

Regional flaps are the transfer of tissue that is near the defect but does not share a common border. An interpolation flap is transposed with the pedicle above or below the native tissue and the distal extent is sutured into the defect as much as possible. Initially, the pedicle provides the blood supply to the flap, but neovascularization occurs with the

Rotation flap

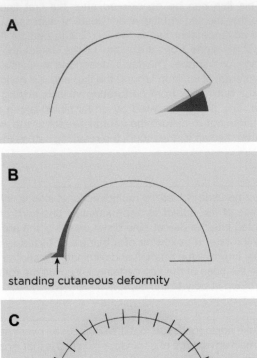

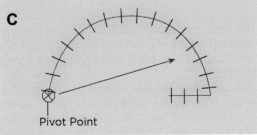

standing cutaneous deformity

Pivot Point

Fig. 3. A. Defect and design of the flap. B. Rotation of the flap. C. Final closure Figure 4-A. Design of the z-plasty. B. Transposition of the flaps and final closure Figure 5-A. Geometric design of the flap. B. Incision and transposition of the flap. C. Final closure.

development of blood vessels from the edge of the defect into the flap. In 14 to 21 days, the ingrowth of blood vessels should be sufficient to divide the pedicle of the flap and finish insetting the remaining flap. The main disadvantage of regional flaps is the need for a second surgery to divide the pedicle and inset the flap.

Distant Flaps

Distant flaps can be transferred from any part of the body and are not limited to a geographic area. The groin flap, supplied by the superficial circumflex iliac artery, involves suturing the defect to the abdominal wall tissue at the inguinal ligament area typically for reconstruction of hand or forearm defects. A cross-leg flap involves raising a flap from the leg contralateral to the defect and suturing the legs together. The pedicle is divided after neovascularization of the flap at the recipient site. These traditional workhorse distant flaps have been supplanted by microvascular free tissue transfer for numerous reasons. Free tissue transfer can be tailored to reconstruct any defect by including a combination of tissue types such as skin, fascia, muscle, tendons, and bone; however, this topic is beyond the scope of this article.

Rhombic transposition flap

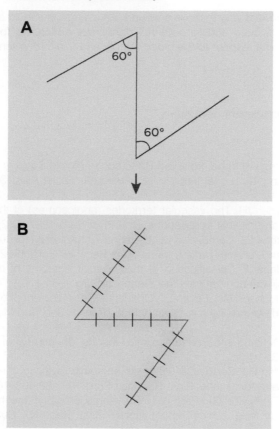

Fig. 4. A Z-plasty lengthens or rearranges a contracted scar by transposing equal lateral limbs over a central limb.

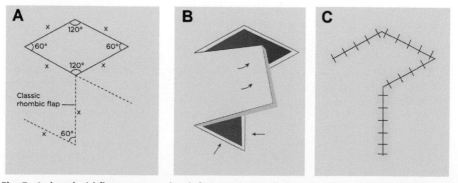

Fig. 5. A rhomboid flap converts the defect into a parallelogram with equal lengths (*x*) and transposes a parallel flap of equal lengths to redirect the tension of closure by 90°.

SUMMARY

There is no one correct way to close a wound but a surgeon should assess the characteristics of the wound and all potential donor site options to formulate a plan. Designing a flap with respect to the blood supply and minimizing tension will lead to success.

DISCLOSURE

The author has no relevant disclosures.

REFERENCES

1. Kayser MR. Surgical flaps. Selected Readings in Plastic Surgery 1999;9(2):1–63.
2. Clark JM, Wang TD. Local flaps in scar revision. Facial Plast Surg 2001;17(4): 295–308.
3. Taylor GI, Palmer JH. The vascular territories (angiosomes) of the body: experimental study and clinical applications. Br J Plast Surg 1987;40(2):113–41.
4. Chang N, Mathes SJ. Comparison of the effect of bacterial inosculation in musculocutaneous and random-pattern flaps. Plast Reconstr Surg 1982;70(1):1–10.
5. Mathes SJ, Nahai F. Classification of the vascular anatomy of muscles: experimental and clinical correlation. Plast Reconstr Surg 1981;67(2):177–87.
6. Heggers JP, Roboson MC, Doran ET. Quantitative assessment of bacterial contamination of open wounds by a slide technique. Trans R Soc Trop Med Hyg 1969;63: 532–4.
7. Heggers JP. Defining infection in chromic wounds: does it matter? J Wound Care 1998;7:389–92.
8. Taylor GI, Corlett RJ, Caddy CM, et al. An anatomic review of the delay phenomenon: II clinical applications. Plast Reconstr Surg 1992;89:408–16.
9. Houseman ND, Taylor GI, Pan WR. The angiosomes of the head and neck: anatomic study and clinical applications. Plast Reconstr Surg 2000;105(7): 2287–313.

Biologic and Synthetic Cellular and/or Tissue-Based Products and Smart Wound Dressings/Coverings

James Abdo, MD, Holly Ortman, MD*

KEYWORDS

- CTP • Graft • Wound treatment • Bioengineered • Burn

KEY POINTS

- Cellular and/or tissue-based products (CTPs) for wounds are becoming more advanced and have revolutionized wound healing by decreasing healing times; providing long-lasting coverage and decreased pain; and decreasing morbidity by replacing lost tissue and increasing the durability, cosmesis, and function of healed wounds.
- There are many products available, making it difficult to select the appropriate one. Products can be characterized as nonviable cells, tissue based, animal; nonviable cells, tissue based, human; viable human cells, cultured in vitro, animal substrate; viable human cells, cultured in vitro, synthetic substrate; viable human cells, noncultured, intact tissue.
- The use of CTPs follows the basic principles of wound care: early excision of nonviable tissue, correction of underlying cause of the wound, treatment of infection, then dressings, closure.
- CTPs need to be closely monitored postapplication for possible complications, including hematoma, separation from the recipient bed, and infection.
- CTPs are a helpful adjunct in preparation of the wound bed and in cases with no available autograft donor sites.

INTRODUCTION

Wound care continues to evolve as advances are made both in the understanding of tissue healing and in materials and technology in the dressings used to treat wounds. The basic principles have changed little since the earliest written records of wound care. In 1650 BC, the Egyptians described a dressing consisting of lint (vegetable fibers), grease, and honey applied to strips of cotton or linen then placed over a wound.[1] The vegetable fibers likely had an absorbent role to help manage drainage,

General Surgery, Marshfield Clinic Health System, 3C1 General Surgery Residency, 1000 North Oak Avenue, Marshfield, WI 54449, USA
* Corresponding author.
E-mail address: ortman.holly@marshfieldclinic.org

Surg Clin N Am 100 (2020) 741–756
https://doi.org/10.1016/j.suc.2020.05.006
0039-6109/20/© 2020 Elsevier Inc. All rights reserved.

the grease consisted of animal fats that likely acted as a barrier to prevent further contamination, and honey has since been found to have antibacterial effects, all of which continue to be important traits of modern wound dressings.[1] The importance of keeping a wound bed moist was first reported in Greek medicine,[1] then eventually proved in clinical trials in the mid–twentieth century.[1-4] This discovery coincided with the advent of new synthetic polymers and fibers. Using new materials dressings could be designed to change the local environment in order to optimize conditions for wound healing. This was a great advancement over the only previously available option: cotton gauze.[1] As new factors are found to influence wound healing such as biofilms and matrix-metalloproteinases (MMPs) dressings that account for these new variables are quick to follow.

The understanding of wound management has led the materials science research in development of cellular and/or tissue-based products (CTPs). Early excision and skin grafting, along with improved critical care management of patients with burns, led to increased survival of patients with greater than 70% total body surface area affected.[6] In such severe cases, there is frequently insufficient donor skin for harvesting autografts to cover the entire burned surface area.[5,6] No CTP has replaced split-thickness skin grafting as the gold standard; however, they remain helpful adjuncts.[6,7] Before the development of bioengineered CTPs, there were only allografts and xenografts available, each of which had their own drawbacks, including allogenicity, harvesting, donor site morbidity, and processing.[8,9] The characteristics of the ideal wound dressing remain largely unchanged since first outlined in the mid-1980s (**Box 1**). The ideal skin substitute has not yet been developed, but both the range and the uses of the CTPs have greatly expanded.

Most current bioengineered CTPs provide temporary closure of the wound and aid in preparation of a neodermal layer, helping prepare the wound bed before

---

Box 1
Properties of an ideal skin substitute

Increase healing

Decrease pain

Are safe

Are cost-effective

Are nonallergenic/nonantigenic/nontoxic

Are easy to apply and remove

Are flexible

Are moisture permeable

Provide an infection barrier

Are durable/resist shearing

Recreate epidermis and dermis

Provide long-term/permanent wound cover

Are easy to manufacture and store

Are easy to obtain/easily available

Have a long shelf life

Data from Refs.[5,10,13,49]

autografting with split-thickness skin grafts for replacement of the epidermal layer. Although initially developed for use in burn injuries, they have found use in acute and chronic wounds because they may require a less vascularized wound bed, increase the dermal component of the healed wound, reduce or remove inhibitory factors, reduce the inflammatory response, and provide rapid and safe coverage.[10] In addition, some newer products have been designed to address specific aspects that may delay or inhibit wound healing.[11–13] Some examples are new antibiotic delivery systems, growth factors, metalloprotease inhibitors, and other substances to counteract factors inhibiting wound healing.[13,14] This article discusses current products on the market and provides information that may aid in choosing the appropriate CTP. An up-to-date list of current available US Food and Drug Administration (FDA)–approved CTPs and so-called smart wound dressings/coverings is shown in **Table 1**.

BIOENGINEERING

The treatment of chronic skin wounds has rapidly accelerated since the 1980s. One of the greatest recent advancements in this healing process is the bioengineering of CTPs. In 2018, Davison-Kolter and colleagues[15] proposed a revised classification system for CTPs that corrected older classification systems, allowing a more intuitive system. This new system uses cellularity, layering, replaced region, materials used, and permanence to organize CTPs. Acellular versus cellular is commonly considered an important factor because this often determines the complexity involved in manufacturing the product. Layering refers to single-layer or bilayer grafts. The region replaced refers to whether the product will be used to replace epidermis, dermis, or both, with bilayer grafts usually used for replacement of the combination of epidermis and dermis.[16] Materials are either natural (eg, cadaveric, amniotic membrane, porcine collagen), synthetic, or both. Permanence (either temporary or permanent CTP's) does not have much bearing as all products to date have temporary components and contain no permanent nonbiodegradable components.[17]

Acellular skin grafts provide a scaffold for wound healing, whereas cellular skin grafts are composed of viable cells indirectly contributing to replacement of lost tissue.[11] Most currently available bioengineered products are acellular and have a variety of sources, including cadaver, amniotic membrane, and porcine or bovine collagen. The acellular scaffold allows host cells (epithelial cells, fibroblasts, and vascular endothelial cells) to migrate into the scaffold, bind, and proliferate.[18]

Cellular-based CTPs include viable cells, such as fibroblasts and/or keratinocytes, that are capable of actively contributing to replacement of lost tissue and are sometimes derived from similar sources as acellular products.[11,16] There are many hurdles that must be overcome when developing a cellular product, one of the greatest being antigenicity. In order to address this, amniotic membrane and neonatal foreskin have been used as sources for cells, which are then placed on a bioabsorbable matrix. These products contain or produce growth factors and stimulate cellular proliferation within the wound bed to support healing.[11] Cellular product use is limited by their high cost and short shelf life.[17] Most require multiple applications in order to achieve adequate wound healing, which also limits use.[11,17]

APPLICATION OF CELLULAR AND/OR TISSUE-BASED PRODUCTS AND WOUND SELECTION

The use of CTPs follows the basic principles of wound healing. Identifying and addressing the underlying wound pathophysiology is essential in maximizing the likelihood of successful application of the CTP.[7,14,19–25] Effective management of any

Table 1
List of graft and smart wound coverings

Graft Trade Name	Manufacturer	Cellularity	Skin Layer	Source Type	Source
Human					
Affinity Human Amniotic Allograft	Organogenesis, Inc, Canton, MA; MTF Biologics	Cellular	Dermal	Amniotic membrane	—
AlloPatch HD Acellular Dermal Matrix	Edison, NJ; MTF Biologics	Acellular	Dermal	Cadaver	—
AlloPatch Pliable AlloSkin AC Acellular Dermal Matrix AlloSkin RT	Edison, NJ; AlloSource, Centennial, CO; AlloSource, Centennial, CO	Acellular Acellular Acellular	Dermal Dermal Dermal	Cadaver Cadaver Cadaver	—
AlloWrap	AlloSource, Centennial, CO	Acellular	Dermal	Amniotic membrane	—
AltiPlasti	Aziyo Biologics, Silver Springs, MD	Acellular	Dermal	Amniotic membrane	—
AltiPly	Aziyo Biologics, Silver Spring, MD	Acellular	Epidermal and dermal	Amniotic membrane	—
AmnioBand Allograft Placental Matrix	MTF Biologics, Edison, NJ	Acellular	Dermal	Amniotic membrane	—
Amnioexcel	Integra LifeSciences Corp acquired Derma Sciences, Plainsboro, NJ	Acellular	Dermal	Amniotic membrane	—
AmnioFill Human Placental Tissue Allograft	MiMex Group, Inc, Marietta, GA	Acellular	Dermal	Amniotic membrane	—
AmnioFix Amnion/Chorion membrane Allograft	MiMex Group, Inc, Marietta, GA	Acellular	Dermal	Amniotic membrane	—
Amniomatrix Human Amniotic Suspension Allograft	Integra LifeSciences Corp acquired Derma Sciences, Plainsboro, NJ	Acellular	Dermal	Amniotic membrane	—
Artacent Wound	Tides Medical, Lafayette, LA	Acellular	Dermal	Amniotic membrane	—

BioDFactor Viable Tissue Matrix	Integra LifeSciences Corp acquired Derma Sciences, Plainsboro, NJ	Acellular	Dermal	Amniotic membrane	—
Biodfence	Integra LifeSciences Corp acquired Derma Sciences, Plainsboro, NJ	Acellular	Dermal	Amniotic membrane	—
Biovance Amniotic membrane Allograft Cellasta Amniotic membrane	Alliqua Biomedical, Langhorne, PA; Ventris Medical, Newport Beach, CA	Acellular Acellular	Dermal Dermal	Amniotic membrane Amniotic membrane	—
Cygnus Amnion Patch Allografts	Vivex Biomedical, Atlanta, GA; HCT/P	Acellular	Dermal	Amniotic membrane	—
Dermacell Human Acellular Dermal Matrix and Dermacell AWM Dermapure	LifeNet Health, Virginia Beach, VA; Tissue Regenix Group, San Antonio, TX	Acellular Acellular	Dermal Dermal	Cadaver Cadaver	—
DermaSpan Acellular Dermal Matrix Dermavest and Plurivest Human Placental Connective Tissue Matr	Zimmer Biomet (manufactured by Biomet Orthopedics, Warsaw, IN) Aedicell, Inc, Honeoye Falls, NY; HCT/P	Acellular Acellular	Dermal Dermal	Cadaver Amniotic membrane	—
Epicord Epicel	MiMedx, Marietta, GA Vericel, Cambridge, MA	Acellular Cellular	Dermal Dermal	Amniotic membrane Cultured epithelial autograft	—
Epifix	MiMedx	Acellular	Dermal	Amniotic membrane	—
FlōGraft Amniotic Fluid-Derived Allograft	Applied Biologics, Scottsdale, AZ	Cellular	Dermal	Amniotic membrane	—
Floweramniopatch and Floweramnioflo	Flower Orthopedics, Horsham, PA	Acellular	Dermal	Amniotic membrane	—

(continued on next page)

Table 1
(continued)

Graft Trade Name	Manufacturer	Cellularity	Skin Layer	Source Type	Source
FlowerDerm	Flower Orthopedics, Horsham, PA;	Acellular	Dermal	Cadaver	—
GammaGraft	Promethean LifeSciences, INC.,	Acellular	Dermal	Cadaver	
Grafix GrafixPL	Pittsburgh, PA; Osiris	Cellular	Dermal	Amniotic membrane	
Prime	Therapeutics, Inc, Columbia, MD	Cellular	Dermal	Amniotic membrane	
GraftJacket RTM	Osiris Therapeutics, Inc, Columbia, MD	Acellular	Dermal	Cadaver	
hMatrix ADM	Wright Medical Group N.V., Memphis, TN	Acellular	Dermal	Cadaver	
	Bacterin International, Inc, Belgrade, MT				
Integra BioFix Amniotic membrane Allograft	Integra LifeSciences	Acellular	Dermal	Amniotic membrane	—
Integra BioFix Flow Placental Tissue Matrix Allograft	Integra LifeSciences	Acellular	Dermal	Amniotic membrane	—
InteguPly	Aziyo Biologics, Silver Springs, MD	Acellular	Dermal	Cadaver	—
Interfyl Human Connective Tissue Matrix	Alliqua Biomedical RTI Surgical, Alachua, FL	Acellular	Dermal	Amniotic membrane	—
Matrix HD Allograft		Acellular	Dermal	Cadaver	
Neox Wound Allografts	Amniox Medical, Inc, Miami, FL	Acellular	Dermal	Amniotic membrane	—
NuShield	Organogenesis, Inc, Canton, MA	Acellular	Dermal	Amniotic membrane	—
PalinGen membrane and Hydromembrane	Amnio Technology LLC, Phoenix, AZ	Acellular	Dermal	Amniotic membrane	—
Revita	StimLabs, LLC, Roswell, GA	Acellular	Dermal	Amniotic membrane	—
LifeNet Health, Virginia Beach, VA (Procurement and processing) Solsys Medical, Newport News, VA					

	Distribution	Cellular	Epidermal and dermal	Cadaver	
TheraSkin					—
WoundEx membrane and WoundEx Flow	Skye Biologics, Inc, El Segundo, CA	Acellular	Dermal	Amniotic membrane	—
Xwrap Amniotic Membrane—derived Allograft	Applied Biologics, Scottsdale, AZ	Acellular	Dermal	Amniotic membrane	—
Animal					
Architect stabilized collagen matrix	Harbor MedTech, Inc, Irvine, CA	Acellular	Dermal	Decellularized equine pericardial tissue	Horse
Bio-ConneKt Wound Matrix CoreLeader Biotech, New Taipei City	MLM Biologics, Inc, Alachua, FL	Acellular	Dermal	Reconstituted collagen derived from equine tendon	Horse
Colla-pad	Taiwan	Acellular	Dermal	Bovine sourced Collagen	Cow
CollaSorb collagen dressing Collamatrix Co, Ltd, Miaoli County	Hartmann USA, Rock Hill, SC	Acellular	Dermal	Bovine sourced Collagen	Cow
CollaWound collagen sponge	Taiwan	Acellular	Dermal	Porcine collagen	Pig
Collexa	Innocoll Pharmaceuticals, Ireland	Acellular	Dermal	Collagen derived from bovine and equine Achilles tendons	Horse/cow
Cytal wound matrix	Acell, Inc, Columbia, MD; United States	Acellular	Dermal	Porcine urinary bladder matrix	Pig
Endoform dermal template	Hollister Wound Care, Libertyville, IL	Acellular	Dermal	Bovine collagen	Cow
Excellagen	Taxus Cardium Pharmaceuticals Group, San Diego, CA	Acellular	Dermal	Bovine dermal collagen	Cow
EZ Derm	Mölnlycke Health Care, Norcross, GA	Acellular	Dermal	Porcine dermis	Pig
Helicoll	EnColl Corp, Fremont, CA	Acellular	Dermal	Bovine collagen	Cow

(continued on next page)

Table 1
(continued)

Bovine Tendon

Graft Trade Name	Manufacturer	Cellularity	Skin Layer	Source Type	Source
Integra LifeSciences Corp, Plainsboro, NJ	—	Acellular	Dermal	Collagen and glycosaminoglycan	Cow
Integra Matrix Wound Dressing; originally Avagen wound dressing, NJ					
Kerecis Omega3 Wound (originally Merigen wound dressing)	Kerecis, Alrington, VA	Acellular	Dermal	Fish dermal matrix composed of fish collagen Porcine urinary bladder matrix	Fish
MicroMatrix	ACell	Acellular	Dermal	Porcine liver	Pig
Miroderm	Miromatrix Medical, Inc, Eden Prairie, MN	Acellular	Dermal	—	Pig
Oasis Wound Matrix	Smith & Nephew, Inc, Fort Worth, TX	Acellular	Dermal	Porcine small intestinal submucosa	Pig
Ologen Collagen Matrix	Aeon Astron Europe BV	Acellular	Dermal	Porcine type I atelocollagen and glycosaminoglycans	Pig
PriMatrix Dermal Repair Scaffold	Integra LifeSciences Corp, Plainsboro, NJ	Acellular	Dermal	Fetal bovine dermis	Cow
Puracol and Puracol Plus Collagen Wound Dressings	Medline Industries, Northfield, IL	Acellular	Dermal	Bovine collagen, porcine intestinal	Cow
PuraPly Antimicrobial (PuraPly AM)	Wound Matrix (formally called Organogenesis, Inc, Canton, MA	Acellular	Dermal	Collagen	Pig

Product	Company/Location	Acellular/Cellular	Dermal	Composition	Source
Marine Polymer Technologies, Inc, Talymed	Burlington, MA	Acellular	Dermal	Fibers of poly-N-acetyl glucosamine isolated from microalgae	Algae
TheraForm Standard/Sheet Absorbable Collagen membrane	Sewon Cellontech Co, Seoul, Korea	Acellular	Dermal	Porcine Collagen	Pig
Synthetic/combination					
Apligraf	Organogenesis, Inc, Canton, MA	Cellular	Dermal	—	Human and animal
Dermagraft	Organogenesis, Inc, Canton, MA	Cellular	Dermal	—	Natural and synthetic
Hyalomatrix tissue reconstruction matrix	Anike Therapeutics, Bedford, MA	Cellular	Dermal	—	Synthetic
Integra Dermal Regeneration Template and Integra Omnigraft Regeneration Template	Integra LifeSciences Corp., Plainsboro, NJ	Acellular	Dermal	Cross-linked bovine tendon collagen and glycosaminoglycan and a semipermeable polysiloxane (silicone layer)	Synthetic and cow
Integra Flowable Wound Matrix	Integra LifeSciences Corp, Plainsboro, NJ	Acellular	Dermal	Granulated cross-linked bovine tendon collagen and glycosaminoglycan and a semipermeable polysiloxane (silicone layer)	Synthetic and cow

(continued on next page)

Table 1
(continued)

Graft Trade Name	Manufacturer	Cellularity	Skin Layer	Source Type	Source
Integra Bilayer Matrix Wound Dressing	Integra LifeSciences Corp, Plainsboro, NJ	Acellular	Dermal	Cross-linked bovine tendon collagen and glycosaminoglycan and a semipermeable polysiloxane (silicone layer)	Synthetic and cow
Restrata	Acera Surgical Inc, St Louis, MO	Acellular	Dermal	—	Synthetic

Abbreviation: HCT/P, human cells, tissues, and cellular and tissue-based products; MTF, Musculoskeletal Transplant Foundation.

acute or chronic wound involves complete removal of nonviable tissue.[22,24,26,27] Infected wounds should be treated and CTPs should not be applied until the infection has resolved.[27] The wound bed should be debrided to tissue with adequate vascular supply to support new tissue growth. Ideally, the wound bed should be uniform and level to ensure maximum contact with the graft. Meticulous hemostasis should be achieved to prevent fluid accumulation or hematoma formation beneath the graft.[22,26,27] Most CTPs are fixed in place with sutures or staples, but some are designed with adhesive intended to adhere around the edges of the wound bed.[28] Some dressings are porous or meshed to allow for fluid egress through the product.[27,28] Coupling these dressings with negative-pressure wound therapy can make postoperative care of the wound easier on both the patient and the provider, with additional benefits including a protective barrier, compression of the graft on the wound minimizing shear and ensuring intimate tissue-graft contact, and continuous removal of excessive fluid from the wound bed while maintaining a moist environment.[27]

Choosing the ideal dressing depends on the structures the wound has disrupted.[20,24,29] Skin is a complex organ composed of epidermal barrier layer, dermal layer giving it structure and elasticity, as well as hair follicles and glands.[30] The depth of injury and, therefore, the structures damaged are often the most important consideration in closure.[30–33] Epidermal injury, characterized by erythema and minor pain, are often caused by sunburns or light scalds and do not require specific surgical treatment. Epidermis regenerates rapidly and without scarring and heals adequately without replacement.[12,20,30]

Superficial partial-thickness wounds affect the epidermis and the superficial parts of the dermis, which can cause epidermal blistering and severe pain. These wounds heal by epithelialization from the margins of the wound (margins can include the wound edge, hair follicles, and sweat gland remnants),[14,32] where basal keratinocytes change into a proliferating migratory cell type and cover the damaged area.[12,14] Complete management of chronic wounds is outside the scope of this article; however, CTPs have become an important tool in management of chronic wounds.[14,16,17,20,21] The next generation of CTPs will be intended not only to replace the dermal and epidermal components but also to replace hair follicles and sebaceous sweat glands.[11,12,33–35]

Deep partial-thickness injuries extend deeper into the dermis and destroy more skin appendages, disrupting dermal structure and increasing healing time.[30] In addition, there is often more pronounced scarring because of more intensive fibroplasia.[12] Application of dermal substitutes can provide excellent protection of the wound, allows regeneration of a vascular bed, can help fill defects and provide smooth surfaces for future skin grafting, as well as preventing pronounced scarring and intensive fibroplasia.[12,14,26,30]

Full-thickness injury refers to injury to the epidermis and the dermis, destroying all epithelial regenerative elements. Full-thickness injuries heal by contraction and epithelialization from only the edge of the wound.[12,17,30] Contraction and fibrosis lead to both cosmetic and functional defects.[36] With loss of the intradermal epithelial regenerative elements, it is impossible to for skin to heal with normal appearance and function.[12,30,36] Full-thickness wounds often have exposed underlying structures, such as fascia, tendon, or even bone.[7,28,30] There are several dermal substitutes available for management of full-thickness wounds.[16,17,37] Integra has been used to cover exposed structures such as bone and tendon and fill in these deep wounds with a vascularized subdermal/dermal-like layer to provide cover, decrease functional morbidity, and improve cosmetic results.[22,23,26,30] All dermal substitutes are designed to provide this vascularized wound bed and need further epidermal covering. Some CTPs are designed to enhance epithelialization from wound edges,[38] but wounds that do not epithelialize from wound edges require epidermal autografts.[14,17,20–22]

After a vascularized neodermis is present, epidermal coverage is needed for final closure of the wound. Split-thickness autografts remain the gold standard of epidermal replacement. Another form of cellular skin graft is the cultured epidermal autograft (CEA). These grafts use the patient's own cells to create the graft. Although CEAs have been used for more than 20 years, use is limited, and at times impractical, because of fragility, cost, time required to produce the graft, and the short shelf life.[39,40] The increased fragility is thought to be related to defective anchoring fibrils in the graft sites.[29,39] These grafts are primarily used in burn injuries.[17] At present, Epicel (Genzyme) is a CEA that is FDA approved to permanently replace epidermis.[41] However, there are several other devices and CEA systems available internationally that are designed to minimize the disadvantages such as shorter culture times.[17] Using a small area of donor skin, keratinocytes are cultured into sheets and attached to petrolatum gauze, which is then sutured into the wound.[29,34,42] Epicel is currently only indicated in patients with deep dermal or full-thickness burns more than 30% or more of affected body surface area or when otherwise unable to use split-thickness autografting.[41]

POSTAPPLICATION CARE

There are many factors that direct care of the CTP after application. Dressings applied in the operating room are determined by the surgeon based on manufacturer recommendations. The wound type is also essential to consider when dressing the wound. The principal of care for venous leg ulcer involves compression. Diabetic foot ulcers require offloading. Avoiding shear forces is essential to allow for neovascularization of the wound bed and to avoid postapplication complications, such as hematoma or seroma formation, which frequently requires replacement of the CTP because it rarely can be salvaged. Physical therapy is often involved postapplication. Range-of-motion exercises should avoid shearing forces to the CTP. Instruction in positioning/transferring methodologies is necessary to protect the product. Negative pressure wound therapy (NPWT) may expedite the wound healing process and allow earlier autograft application as well as increase the take of the CTP.[22]

For bilayered living cellular constructs (eg, Apligraf), the dressing must be kept dry until the follow-up appointment, and, at day 7, the secondary dressing alone is removed for wound inspection and evaluation with the primary dressing left undisturbed; the secondary dressing is then reapplied. On postoperative day 14, both dressings are removed, followed by a light normal saline wash and avoidance of any debridement or wound bed disturbance. New primary and secondary dressings are then applied, and this process of replacing primary and secondary dressings to monitor wound healing is performed on a weekly basis with reapplication of Apligraf performed if needed.[19] Dermal replacement matrix (eg, Integra Bilayer Wound Matrix) involves a fixation layer (elastic net dressing), compression layer, bulky dressing layer, optional antishear layer, and antimicrobial layer with splints or bolsters for the first 5 to 7 days; NPWT may be used for mesh graft sites as well. Dressing changes are then performed every 2 to 3 days.[19,43] All dressings, with the exception of the elastic net dressing, are removed to inspect. The antimicrobial dressing is remoistened every 6 to 8 hours, or more as needed, and changed every 3 days.[19,43] Shear forces are minimized and pressure avoided. Range-of-motion exercises may begin on postoperative day 5 to 7.[43] The silicone layer overlying the neodermis is typically ready for removal around postoperative day 21, followed by application of the autograft.[43] Acellular dermal matrix (eg, Alloderm) is dressed in 3 layers: petrolatum-based antimicrobial impregnated gauze, damp saline gauze, and outer layer of dry gauze with an elastic bandage.[43] The outer 2 layers are replaced as often as necessary, but the innermost layer is not changed until postoperative day 7.[43]

Postapplication care is directed toward the most common causes of product failure, including hematoma, fluid accumulation, purulence/infection, and incomplete adherence or detachment caused by mechanical forces. If complications are avoided, and appropriate granulation tissue forms, a split-thickness skin graft may be applied with a failure rate of only 7%, which is lower than after applying an autograft directly on tendons with or without granulation tissue.[44,45]

The ideal CTP has not yet been developed; it would be safe and stable, and would have the characteristics of excellent adherence, control of moisture permeability, infection control, adequate pain control, appropriate transparency, cost-effectiveness, and relative ease of application and removal[46] (see **Box 1**).

Current avenues of research include different sources for CTP derivatives, more complex CTPs, and various methodologies to create the ideal CTP. Research is investigating different species for derivation of CTP products. Collagen peptides from the jellyfish *Rhopilema esculentum* have been found to be able to accelerate wound healing with re-epithelialization, tissue regeneration, and increased collagen deposition.[47] Research is also underway on types of synthetic, biologic, and complex CTP development. Smart trilayer (epidermis, dermis, and hypodermis) CTPs are also being investigated for efficient deep wound healing and have been found to have improved and expedited wound healing in vivo.[48] Another area of research is three-dimensional (3D) printing. This technology is being developed to regenerate tissues and organs for transplant. It allows mimicking and fabrication of skin on a 3D scaffold with cells from skin cell lines and human mesenchymal stem cells without negative effect.

SUMMARY

The core tenets of wound healing have not changed and should continue to be followed. Only when the wound has been adequately debrided, underlying causes have been identified and treated, and all infection has cleared should the clinician consider options to close the wound. For replacement of the epidermis, split-thickness skin grafting remains the gold standard. There are many options for permanent/semi-permanent wound coverings, with new bioengineered options being developed frequently. Many of these dressings are designed to be used in conjunction with split-thickness skin grafting. The key to choosing the appropriate dressing is replacing the tissue lost.[30] Many dermal substitutes can help with early neovascularization of the wound bed to support epithelial in-growth.[16] The benefits of CTPs have been established, and CTPs represent the vanguard of regenerative medicine and continue to make contributions to many other fields of medicine.

DISCLOSURE

The authors have nothing to disclose.

REFERENCES

1. Ovington L. The art and science of wound dressings in the twenty-first century. In: Falabella A, Kirsner R, editors. Wound healing. Boca Raton (FL): Taylor & Francis; 2005. p. 587–98.

2. Gilje O. Ulcus cruris in venous circulatory disturbances. Investigations of the etiology, pathogenesis and therapy of leg ulcers. (Thesis). Acta Derm Venerol 1949; 22:159–74.

3. Winter GD. Formation of the scab and the rate of epithelization of superficial wounds in the skin of the young domestic pig. Nature 1962;193(4812):293–4.

4. Winter GD. Effect of air exposure and occlusion on experimental human skin wounds. Nature 1963;200(4904):378–9.

5. Sheridan RL, Tompkins RG. Skin substitutes in burns. Burns 1999;25(2):97–103.

6. Herndon DN. Total burn care. Philadelphia: Elsevier Health Sciences; 2007.

7. Rowan MP, Cancio LC, Elster EA, et al. Burn wound healing and treatment: review and advancements. Crit Care 2015;19(1):243.

8. Hermans MHE. Preservation methods of allografts and their (lack of) influence on clinical results in partial thickness burns. Burns 2011;37(5):873–81.

9. Hermans MHE. Porcine xenografts vs. (cryopreserved) allografts in the management of partial thickness burns: Is there a clinical difference? Burns 2014;40(3): 408–15.

10. Shores JT, Gabriel A, Gupta S. Skin substitutes and alternatives: a review. Adv Skin Wound Care 2007;20(9):493.

11. Miller J, Wynes J. Updates on bioengineered alternative tissues. Clin Podiatr Med Surg 2019;36(3):413–24.

12. Shevchenko RV, James SL, James SE. A review of tissue-engineered skin bioconstructs available for skin reconstruction. J R Soc Interface 2010;7(43):229–58.

13. Límová M. Active wound coverings: bioengineered skin and dermal substitutes. Surg Clin North Am 2010;90(6):1237–55.

14. Woo K, Ayello EA, Sibbald RG. The edge effect: current therapeutic options to advance the wound edge. Adv Skin Wound Care 2007;20(2):99.

15. Davison-Kotler E, Sharma V, Kang NV, et al. A universal classification system of skin substitutes inspired by factorial design. Tissue Eng Part B Rev 2018;24(4): 279–88.

16. Snyder D, Sullivan N, Margolis D. Skin substitutes for treating chronic wounds. Agency for Healthcare Research and Quality (US) 2020. Available at: http://www.ncbi.nlm.nih.gov/books/NBK554220/. Accessed June 4, 2020.

17. Dai C, Shih S, Khachemoune A. Skin substitutes for acute and chronic wound healing: an updated review. J Dermatol Treat 2018;0(ja):1–33.

18. Alavii A, Kirsner RS. Dressings. In: Bolognia JL, Schaffer JV, Cerroni L, editors. Dermatology. 4th edition. China: Elsevier; 2017. p. 2462–77.

19. How is Apligraf® applied?. Available at: http://www.apligraf.com/patient/what_is_apligraf/how_is_apligraf_applied.html. Accessed December 17, 2019.

20. Powers JG, Higham C, Broussard K, et al. Wound healing and treating wounds: Chronic wound care and management. J Am Acad Dermatol 2016;74(4):607–25.

21. Frykberg RG, Banks J. Challenges in the treatment of chronic wounds. Adv Wound Care 2015;4(9):560–82.

22. Jeschke MG, Rose C, Angele P, et al. Development of new reconstructive techniques: use of integra in combination with fibrin glue and negative-pressure therapy for reconstruction of acute and chronic wounds. Plast Reconstr Surg 2004; 113(2):525.

23. Buchanan PJ, Kung TA, Cederna PS. Evidence-based medicine: wound closure. Plast Reconstr Surg 2016;138(3S):257S.

24. Fonder MA, Lazarus GS, Cowan DA, et al. Treating the chronic wound: A practical approach to the care of nonhealing wounds and wound care dressings. J Am Acad Dermatol 2008;58(2):185–206.

25. Schultz GS, Barillo DJ, Mozingo DW, et al. Wound bed preparation and a brief history of TIME. Int Wound J 2004;1(1):19–32.

26. Fitton AR, Drew P, Dickson WA. The use of a bilaminate artificial skin substitute (IntegraTM) in acute resurfacing of burns: an early experience. Br J Plast Surg 2001;54(3):208–12.

27. INTEGRA™ Meshed Bilayer Wound Matrix - Product Description and Benefits. Available at: http://www.ilstraining.com/IMBWM/imbwm/imbwm_it_01.html. Accessed December 12, 2019.

28. Abdel-Sayed P, Hirt-Burri N, de Buys Roessingh A, et al. Evolution of Biological Bandages as First Cover for Burn Patients. Adv Wound Care (New Rochelle) 2019;8(11):555–64.

29. Broussard KC, Powers JG. Wound dressings: selecting the most appropriate type. Am J Clin Dermatol 2013;14(6):449–59.

30. Papini R. Management of burn injuries of various depths. BMJ 2004;329(7458): 158–60.

31. van der Veen VC, van der Wal MBA, van Leeuwen MCE, et al. Biological background of dermal substitutes. Burns 2010;36(3):305–21.

32. Roger M, Fullard N, Costello L, et al. Bioengineering the microanatomy of human skin. J Anat 2019;234(4):438–55.

33. Augustine R, Kalarikkal N, Thomas S. Advancement of wound care from grafts to bioengineered smart skin substitutes. Prog Biomater 2014;3(2):103–13.

34. Ehrenreich M, Ruszczak Z. Update on tissue-engineered biological dressings. Tissue Eng 2006;12(9):2407–24.

35. Lu G, Huang S. Bioengineered CTPs: key elements and novel design for biomedical applications. Int Wound J 2013;10(4):365–71.

36. Halim AS, Khoo TL, Mohd. Yussof, et al. Biologic and synthetic skin substitutes: An overview. Indian J Plast Surg 2010;43(Suppl):S23–8.

37. Rehim SA, Singhal M, Chung KC. Dermal CTPs for upper limb reconstruction: current status, indications, and contraindications. Hand Clin 2014;30(2):239–52.

38. Lesher AP, Curry RH, Evans J, et al. Effectiveness of Biobrane for treatment of partial-thickness burns in children. J Pediatr Surg 2011;46(9):1759–63.

39. Woodley DT, Peterson HD, Herzog SR, et al. Burn wounds resurfaced by cultured epidermal autografts show abnormal reconstitution of anchoring fibrils. JAMA 1988;259(17):2566–71.

40. Sood R, Roggy D, Zieger M, et al. Cultured epithelial autografts for coverage of large burn wounds in eighty-eight patients: the indiana university experience. J Burn Care Res 2010;31(4):559–68.

41. Research C for BE and. Epicel (cultured epidermal autografts). FDA. 2019. Available at: http://www.fda.gov/vaccines-blood-biologics/approved-blood-products/ epicel-cultured-epidermal-autografts. Accessed December 17, 2019.

42. Rheinwald JG, Green H. Formation of a keratinizing epithelium in culture by a cloned cell line derived from a teratoma. Cell 1975;6(3):317–30.

43. Integra LifeSciences. Integra Treatment Guidelines. INTEGRA● Bilayer Matrix Wound Dressing - Product Brochures, Letters and Inserts. 2017. Available at: http://www.ilstraining.com/bmwd/brochures.html. Accessed June 5, 2020.

44. Yeong E-K, Yu Y-C, Chan Z-H, et al. Is artificial dermis an effective tool in the treatment of tendon-exposed wounds? J Burn Care Res 2013;34(1):161–7.

45. Donegan, R. J., Schmidt, B. M., & Blume, P. A. (2014). An overview of factors maximizing successful split-thickness skin grafting in diabetic wounds. Diabetic Foot & Ankle, 5, 10.3402/dfa.v5.24769. https://doi.org/10.3402/dfa.v5.24769

46. Woodroof EA. The Search for an Ideal Temporary skin substitute: AWBAT. Eplasty 2009;9:95–104. Available at: https://www.ncbi.nlm.nih.gov/pmc/articles/PMC2643124/. Accessed December 17, 2019.

47. Felician FF, Yu R-H, Li M-Z, et al. The wound healing potential of collagen peptides derived from the jellyfish Rhopilema esculentum. Chin J Traumatol 2019; 22(1):12–20.

48. Haldar S, Sharma A, Gupta S, et al. Bioengineered smart trilayer skin tissue substitute for efficient deep wound healing. Mater Sci Eng C Mater Biol Appl 2019; 105:110140.

49. Pruitt BA, Levine NS. Characteristics and uses of biologic dressings and skin substitutes. Arch Surg 1984;119(3):312–22.

Bacteria and Antibiotics in Wound Healing

Michael D. Caldwell, MD, PhD, FACS

KEYWORDS

- Bacteria • Antibiotics • Tissue repair

KEY POINTS

- Microbes delay repair. Persistent microbial flora leads to persistent inflammation.
- Microbial flora can direct persistence or lysis of wound neutrophils.
- This lack of neutrophil apoptosis and/or neutrophil lysis, along with persistent PAMPs/DAMPs, impaired neutrophil apoptosis/efferocytosis, lack of M1-M2 macrophage conversion, results in persistence of the inflammatory stage and the loss of transition to the proliferation stage of repair.

UNITED STATES POPULATION BURDEN OF WOUNDS AND WOUND INFECTIONS

In the first comprehensive study of Medicare spending in wound care, based on retrospective analysis of the 2014 Medicare 5% Limited Data Set for acute and chronic wounds, it was identified that 14.5% or approximately 8.2 million Medicare beneficiaries had at least 1 type of wound or wound-related infection. The largest category were surgical infections (4%), then diabetic wound infection (3.4%), and nonhealing surgical wounds (3.0%). The total Medicare spending estimates for all wound types range from $28.1 billion to $96.8 billion, primarily in the outpatient setting.[1] As the population ages and with the increase in the diabetic population (9.4% of the US population in 2015), it is not surprising that the global burden of wounds and wound infections is rapidly increasing.[2]

HISTORICAL PERSPECTIVE REGARDING BACTERIA AND WOUND HEALING

It was reported in the Edwin Smith Papyrus of 1600 BC that there were two major factors that interfered with wound healing. These were movement with continued trauma to the wound, and suppuration.[3] However, from the time of Hippocrates, suppuration, or pus formation, was thought to be beneficial. With regard to wound healing, Hippocrates wrote that, "if the pus is white and not offensive, health will follow" but "if it is sanious and muddy, death is to be looked for."[4,5] This belief led to the concept of

Center for Hyperbaric Medicine and Tissue Repair, Marshfield Clinic, 1000 North Oak Avenue, Marshfield, WI 54449, USA
E-mail address: caldwell.michael@marshfieldclinic.org

Surg Clin N Am 100 (2020) 757–776
https://doi.org/10.1016/j.suc.2020.05.007
0039-6109/20/© 2020 Elsevier Inc. All rights reserved.

"good and laudable pus" as being important for wound healing. Galen is generally credited with the perpetuation of this concept. However, a close reading of his writings shows that Galen did not believe pus was required for wound healing.[5]

The concept of laudable pus was challenged in the thirteenth century by Theodoric Bourgognoni's call to prevent suppuration to aid in the healing of wounds. This work was supported by that of Henri de Mondeville in the early fourteenth century.[5] However, it was not until the nineteenth century, with the revelations of Semmelweis, Pasteur, and Lister regarding germ theory and antiseptic technique, that the concept of laudable pus was finally discredited and infection control was recognized not only as an aid to healing wounds but to survival after surgery.[6]

The human body exists in a close, normally symbiotic, relationship with bacteria. Infection follows when the relationship is upset by a decrease in host resistance or an increase in bacterial number or virulence. Destruction of the keratin layer of the skin, localized ischemia, or presence of a penetrating foreign body may result in impaired local immunocompetence. Manifestations of attempted localized immune control include cellulitis and abscess formation.[7] A chronic local attempt at control of microbial invasion frequently manifests as a nonhealing wound. As Tarmuzzer and Schulz[8] proposed, wound chronicity begins with bacteria.[8,9]

In 1916, in the first of his extensive series of articles on the cicatrization of wounds, Carrell[10] evaluated the effect of bacteria on wound healing. Carrell and Hartmann took serial wound measurements and cultures every 4 days in injured soldiers. When bacteria were found, the wounds were treated with 0.5% Dakin or 0.2% paratoluene sodium sulfochloramide solutions. They stated, "the regularity of cicatrization depends in a large measure on the bacteriologic conditions of the wound."[10]

The idea then evolved that the magnitude of bacterial inoculation is another factor that can influence the onset of wound infection or impaired wound healing.[7] The first correlation of the quantity of bacteria affecting the risk of infection was made by World War I French surgeons. If battle wounds were more than 15 hours old, the wound was debrided, a culture was taken, irrigation was performed with Dakin solution, and the wound was packed with flavine gauze. On arrival at the base hospital, if there were no streptococci on the culture plate, and if other organisms grew fewer than 5 colonies per culture plate, the wound was closed. If there were any Streptococci or more than 5 colonies of other bacteria, the wound was left to heal by secondary intention. This approach recognized species differences in virulence and was the first documentation of quantitative evaluation of the bacterial contamination of the wound.[7,11]

By World War II, preliminary wound cultures had become part of the standard of care of battle wounds.[12] Howe noted that, once a postoperative infected wound had been converted to a clean wound, it could be closed surgically.[13,14] In the 1950s, surgical decision making shifted from qualitative to quantitative bacteriology. Liedburg and colleagues[15] showed that inoculation of greater than 10^5/mL Streptococci, Pseudomonas, or Staphylococcus aureus in rabbit graft sites destroyed the skin grafts, reducing the graft take from 91% to 32%. Streptococci were twice as deleterious to graft destruction when quantitatively compared with Staphylococci or Pseudomonas. In 1964, Bendy and colleagues,[16] in a prospective clinical trial of patients with decubitus ulcers, produced evidence that suppression of growth of bacterial pathogens was the decisive factor in the healing of decubiti and that topical gentamicin, as a representative broad-spectrum antimicrobial, enhanced this effect. Krizek and colleagues[17] showed decreased full thickness skin autograft survival in experimental animals when the graft bed was immediately inoculated with varying numbers of Pseudomonas aeruginosa, Escherichia coli, or S aureus. They found that 100% of uninfected control animals and grafts survived. However, the mortalities were 68%,

45%, and 55%, and the graft losses were 100%, 60%, and 85% with *Pseudomonas, E coli*, or *Staphylococcus* inoculations, respectively. These investigators correlated their findings with 50 consecutive granulating human wounds. Before skin grafting, serial quantitative bacterial cultures were performed on biopsy specimens during treatment with a variety of topical agents. Irrespective of the type of therapy used, or the specific bacterial flora present, a bacterial level of 10^5 or fewer bacteria per gram of tissue in the wound at the time of surgery was associated with an average graft survival of 93%. In wounds containing greater than 10^5 bacteria per gram of tissue at the time of grafting, the average graft survival was less than 20%.[17] In 1968, Robson and colleagues[18] applied the findings of Krizek and colleaues[17] to delayed wound closure. They retrospectively found that 93% of delayed closures proceeded to uncomplicated healing when the granulation tissue in the incision contained 10^5 or fewer bacteria per gram of tissue at the time of closure. In contrast, all wounds containing greater than 10^5 bacteria per gram of tissue failed delayed closure.[18] Robson and Heggers[19] followed this finding with a prospective study in 95 patients with delayed wound closures in which they found a 96% successful closure rate when the bacterial wound estimate was 10^5 bacteria or fewer per gram of tissue. Robson and colleagues[16] evaluated Howe's conclusions with 94 incisional abscesses of significant size. One group (n = 44) was debrided and allowed to heal by secondary intention (22.3 days of hospitalization) and a subsequent group (n = 50) were closed with delayed closure after determining that the wound bacterial count was 10^5 or fewer (8 days of hospitalization; $P<.01$). Ninety-one percent of the delayed closure group healed without complication. Ninety-three percent of the secondary intention group were not healed at the time of discharge and required further outpatient care.[16] Using heavily contaminated experimental wounds containing 10^6 bacteria per gram of tissue, the effect of microbial contamination on musculocutaneous and random flaps was examined by Murphy in 1970.[20] Neither type of flap was able to prevent bacterial growth and all flaps dehisced. In minimally contaminated wounds containing 10^4 or fewer bacteria, random and musculocutaneous flaps healed accompanied by a decrease in the bacterial level in the wound. In an intermediate group containing 10^5 bacteria per gram of tissue, musculocutaneous flaps reduced the bacterial count and healed, but the random flaps did not control bacterial growth and failed.[20] Breidenbach and Trager,[21] studying complex wounds of the extremities closed with free flaps, found that intraoperative bacterial burden of 10^4 or greater resulted in an 89% postoperative infection rate, whereas an intraoperative bacterial level at less than 10^4 was associated with only a 5% postoperative infection rate.

Following reconstructive vascular surgery in 63 patients with nonhealing ischemic ulcerations, skin grafts were performed on the 55 patients with ankle brachial index greater than 0.47 to reduce the time of ulcer healing. Primary healing of ulcers covered with skin grafts was achieved in 44 of the 55 patients (80%). The difference in healing versus failure of the skin grafts directly correlated with quantitative bacterial counts of more than 5×10^4 colony-forming units (CFU)/cm^2.[22] Høgsberg and colleagues,[23] in a study of 82 consecutive patients with chronic venous leg ulcers, evaluated microbiology, demographic data, smoking and drinking habits, diabetes, renal impairment, comorbidities, approximated size and age of wounds, immunosuppressive treatment, and complicating factors on the clinical outcome of each patient. A logistic regression analysis revealed that the presence of *P aeruginosa* was the sole predictor of healing at 12 weeks. If *Pseudomonas* was present, only 33.3% of split-thickness skin-grafted ulcers healed, whereas 73.1% of ulcers without *Pseudomonas*, healed.[23] Xu and colleagues[24] quantitatively evaluated the microbial concentrations in wound fluid collected from 32 diabetic patients with neuropathic foot ulcers and correlated those findings with change in daily ulcer area. Their study revealed an inverse relationship between wound bioburden and wound healing rate. Specifically, they found that, for each log_{10} order of CFU increase, ulcer healing was delayed by 44%. In those individuals with CFU greater than 10^4 CFU/mL, there was either no change or an increase in wound area during the 28 days of the study.[24] Similar outcomes were found by Lookingbill and colleagues[25] and Daltrey and colleagues.[26]

An important factor in the failure of these wounds to heal is the precedent of polymicrobial flora living cooperatively in highly organized biofilms. These biofilms shield pathogenic microbes from antimicrobial therapy and from the patient's immune response. Biofilm infections have been linked to wound chronicity and it has been shown that biofilm infection may directly hinder wound closure or cause defective closure because of resultant impaired skin barrier function[2] (discussed later).

MECHANISMS FOR MICROBIAL INTERFERENCE WITH WOUND HEALING

The cellular response that results in tissue repair is ordered with regulated intercellular communication. Tissue repair is frequently depicted as consecutive, congruous phases: hemostasis, inflammation, proliferation and remodeling. Dysregulation of this ordered cellular process results in impaired healing, manifesting as chronic nonhealing wounds, excessive scarring, or tumor formation.[27] Two major causes for this dysregulation are the interactions of the innate immune system with repetitive injury and microbial invasion. According to classic immunology, the human immune system is composed of innate and adaptive immunity. The inherited, innate immune system is responsible for a rapid, initial, nonspecific defense response to any foreign body. Key components of this system include leukocytes, dendritic cells, natural killer cells, and complement plasma proteins. The adaptive immune response is responsible for development of memorized, antigen-specific immune responses to specific pathogens. This system contains B cells, T cells, and a memory bank of antigens for easier recognition and attack on pathogens at subsequent exposure. This article concentrates on the interactions of the innate immune system in the repair process.

The innate immune system is considered the first-line host defense system. Its rapid response is crucial in eliminating the spread of infection from the site of injury. Because of its nonspecific nature, the innate immune system relies on recognition of highly conserved molecules of microorganisms and molecules associated with cell injury. The major mediators for cell injury or microbial invasion are, respectively, damage-associated molecular patterns (DAMPs) and pathogen-associated molecular patterns (PAMPs) from invading bacteria, fungi, or viruses. Following cellular stress, inflammation, or necrosis, DAMPs are formed from the release of cytosolic and nuclear proteins, DNA, RNA, and purine metabolites. PAMPs are molecules formed from bacteria, fungi, and viruses present on the skin surface and in the environment. Examples of PAMPs include lipopolysaccharide, lipopeptides, mannose, microbial DNA, double-stranded RNA, flagellin, peptidoglycans, lipoteichoic acid, N-formylmethionine, and lipoprotein.[28,29]

These associated molecular patterns interact with a class of receptors called pattern recognition receptors (PRRs). These PRRs, which allow an immediate immune response, are constitutively expressed on host macrophages, monocytes, dendritic cells, neutrophils, and epithelial cells.[28,29]

The Toll-like receptors (TLRs) represent the first and best-characterized PRR family. Others include the C-type lectin receptors, retinoic acid–inducible gene-I–like receptors (RLR), NOD-like receptors (NLR), AIM2-like receptors (ALR), and intracellular DNA sensors. PRRs activate downstream signaling cascades that lead to situation-specific host immune responses after bacterial, fungal, and viral infections and skin injury. Stimulation of the TLRs through intracellular signaling from adapter proteins leads to nuclear translocation of nuclear factor (NF)-κB, which, in association with mitogen-activated protein kinases, initiates transcription of various inflammatory cytokines, chemokines, antimicrobial peptides, and costimulatory factors.[30]

With the danger signal (DAMPs) initiated, downstream cascades create the inflammatory phase of tissue repair. As the result, cells are stimulated to migrate to the injured site to assist the innate immune response and begin the ordered cellular inflammatory response that leads to repair. This inflammatory phase is highly regulated, and prolongation of the inflammatory phase leads to a chronic nonhealing wound. Neutrophils are the first inflammatory leukocytes recruited to the wound. Under the influence of chemokines, there is a concomitant increased expression of adhesion molecules (ICAM, VCAM1, e-selectin) on vascular endothelial cells, which leads to adherence of neutrophils to vessel walls, then extravasation and migration along a chemokine gradient. This neutrophil migration is accompanied by phagocytosis, killing of engulfed bacteria, release of proteinases and antimicrobial cationic peptides, and production of tumor necrosis factor (TNF)-α, interleukin (IL)-1β, and IL-6, which maintain the inflammatory state.[28,29,31,32]

Neutrophils are the principal cellular defense against bacterial and fungal infections. At sites of infection, neutrophils phagocytose microbes, which in turn are killed by reactive oxygen species (ROS) and neutrophil-elicited antimicrobial peptides (AMPs) and proteases.[31,32] Many of these microbicidal molecules are also cytotoxic to host tissues, and thus release of these molecules from the death of neutrophils can contribute to tissue necrosis and impairment of normal tissue functions such as wound healing.[31] There is normally extensive turnover of neutrophils daily. The interaction of neutrophils with microbes and molecules produced by microbes affects neutrophil turnover.[31] The effects of microbes on neutrophils are frequently microbe specific and can vary from prolonging the life of neutrophils, to stimulating programmed neutrophil death (apoptosis), to neutrophil lysis (oncosis).[33-35] Under normal repair conditions, neutrophils within the wound are removed through a combination of apoptosis and macrophage phagocytosis of the apoptotic neutrophil (efferocytosis).[28,36-42] This process results in containment of the cytotoxic elements that would otherwise be released into the wound in the event of neutrophil oncosis.[28]

Wound macrophages are the key regulators of tissue repair.[36,43] About 3 days after injury, monocyte levels peak as the second class of inflammatory cells recruited into the wound. Monocytes are recruited by the same mechanism involved in neutrophil recruitment, and the response to damage and PAMPs leads to monocyte differentiation into classically (M1) activated macrophages.[44] Wound macrophages can be described as having two general types of activities: M1 macrophages are observed in initial tissue damage/microbial invasion responses. They show increased phagocytosis and proinflammatory cytokine production, which facilitates innate immunity and wound debridement. Alternatively activated, M2 macrophages predominate later in repair; express vascular endothelial cell growth factor, transforming growth factor beta, and IL-10; are activated by varied stimuli; assist in the resolution of inflammation; and promote tissue formation and remodeling.[31,43,45] This M1/M2 polarization of macrophages within the wound has been termed the M1 kill/M2 heal macrophage dichotomy.[46] The conversion of M1 to M2 macrophages is critical to the resolution of the inflammatory phase of tissue repair.[45]

In normal tissue repair, the inflammatory phase is self-limiting. The ratio of classic or alternatively activated wound macrophage phenotypes changes as the wound heals.[45,47] In the early inflammatory response, 85% of macrophages have an M1 phenotype, which release proinflammatory mediators, whereas 15% have an M2 phenotype, which produce antiinflammatory cytokines and growth factors. As the wound matures, only 15% to 20% of macrophages have an M1 phenotype and the wound macrophage population primarily has an M2 phenotype.[45,47,48] Lack of resolution of the inflammatory phase at the site of injury and the typical shift from the M1 to M2 macrophage phenotype characterizes a chronic nonhealing wound.[45,49] Chronic wounds are known to have an abundance of M1 macrophages. At the chronic wound margin, approximately 80% of cells are proinflammatory M1 macrophages.[44,45,50,51] Reduced M2 macrophage levels in diabetic wounds result in a reduction in transforming growth factor β1, insulinlike growth factor-1, and vascular endothelial growth factor, which regulate the proliferative stage of repair.[45] The result of a prolonged inflammatory state is high levels of proinflammatory mediators, such as TNF, IL-1β, IL-17, and inducible nitric oxide synthase and impaired repair.[45] Patients with chronic wounds also present with high levels of proinflammatory cytokines in their wound fluid.[45,50] High levels of proinflammatory mediators, such as TNF, lead to alterations in the balance between matrix metallopeptidases (MMPs) and tissue inhibitor of metalloproteinases, leading to excessive extracellular matrix proteolysis, which contributes to wound chronicity[45] (see the Stephanie R. Goldberg and Robert F. Diegelmann's article, "What Makes Wounds Chronic," in this issue).

The efferocytosis of apoptotic neutrophils is instrumental in the conversion of M1 to M2 macrophages and is a prerequisite for resolution of inflammation in the wound[29,36,45,51] (reviewed in Ref.[28]). Shortly after injury, neutrophils enter the wound and, after clearing microbes and debris, undergo apoptosis. These effete neutrophils are removed by macrophages, which in turn leads to macrophage conversion to the antiinflammatory M2 phenotype. Alterations in the wound environment and impaired efferocytosis can result in persistence of the proinflammatory M1 phenotype, which prolongs inflammation and impairs tissue repair.[28]

Efferocytosis can be altered by abnormalities in macrophage or neutrophil function. Macrophages in chronic wounds have a reduced capacity to phagocytose dead neutrophils. Diabetic patients have macrophages with reduced apoptotic clearance activity caused by hyperglycemia and advanced glycation end products.[45] In patients with chronic venous ulcers, high levels of iron from engulfed erythrocytes in wound macrophages lead to a predominance of the M1 macrophage phenotype and a prolonged inflammatory phase with delayed repair[45,50] (**Fig. 1**).

Effect of Microbes on Neutrophil Function and Resolution of Inflammation

As stated, the resolution of inflammation relies on downregulating neutrophil function, the promotion of neutrophil apoptosis, and then successful clearance of these cells by macrophages. Neutrophil function can be affected by microbial invasion at the level of neutrophil recruitment, phagocytosis, bactericidal activity, and neutrophil apoptosis.

Most neutrophils present within the wound are recruited from blood through extravasation. Some bacteria dampen neutrophil recruitment. *Streptococcus pyogenes* and *Streptococcus pneumoniae* produce factors that target the actions of chemoattractants. *S aureus* and gram-negative pathogens produce molecules that impair chemotaxis and neutrophil extravasation.[52] Neutrophil phagocytosis of bacterial and fungal pathogens is initiated by the recognition of invading microbial pathogens through receptors present on the neutrophil surface, such as TLRs and opsonic receptors, which recognize host proteins that coat the microbial surface.[52] The ligation of PRRs results

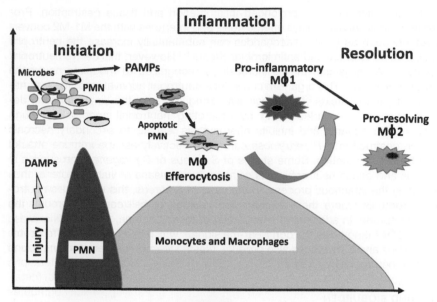

Efferocytosis is a Major Factor in the Conversion from M1 to M2 Phenotype and Resolution of Inflammation

Fig. 1. Neutrophil apoptosis and macrophage phagocytosis of effete neutrophils (efferocytosis) is critical to the resolution of the inflammatory phase of tissue repair and allows the progression of the repair process.

in the production of a complex series of molecular signals that regulate enhanced phagocytosis, microbial killing, and the modulation of inflammation by cytokine production (discussed earlier). Bacterial pathogens (*Streptococcus* spp, *Neisseria meningitidis*, *Klebsiella* spp, *E coli*, *P aeruginosa*, *Haemophilus influenzae*) can mask surface antigens by expressing a polysaccharide capsule that inhibits neutrophil phagocytosis, or structurally modify surface antigens to prevent recognition by PRRs (*Yersinia* spp, *Salmonella typhimurium*).[52] The potent antimicrobial activity of the neutrophil requires the conflation of proteolytic and degradative enzymes, cationic molecules, and ROS. Several bacterial pathogens can either inhibit ROS production or direct the oxidative complex away from the phagosome (*Anaplasma phagocytophilium*, *Francisella tularensis*, *Neisseria gonorrhoeae*, *Helicobacter pylori*, *Yersinia*, *P aeruginosa*). Bacterial pathogens (both gram-positive and gram-negative bacteria) can escape the actions of cationic AMPs by alteration of the surface charge with cationic molecules, thus promoting electrostatic repulsion from the AMPs. In addition, bacterial proteases can inactivate AMPs (*S aureus*, *Proteus mirabilis*, *S pyogenes*, *P aeruginosa*, *Enterococcus faecalis*).[52]

Phagocytosis of microorganisms primes the neutrophil to undergo apoptosis, a response that has been termed phagocytosis-induced cell death.[53] Under normal circumstances, bacterial pathogens such as *E coli*, *P aeruginosa*, and *S aureus* induce neutrophil apoptosis following phagocytosis. The subsequent clearance of apoptotic neutrophils by efferocytosis not only prevents collateral tissue damage but also provides an additional opportunity for pathogen destruction. However, there are certain microbes that can inhibit or delay apoptosis or cause neutrophil lysis (oncosis/

necroptosis), which leads to prolonged inflammation and tissue destruction. Prolonged neutrophil survival delays efferocytosis and interferes with the M1-M2 conversion. Agents such as lipopolysaccharides can substantially increase the neutrophil lifespan, leading to enhanced antimicrobial effects.[53] However, this delays neutrophil efferocytosis. An organism that is increasingly recognized to modulate neutrophil apoptosis is *S aureus*. This organism can induce neutrophil survival, apoptosis, or necrosis in different contexts.[53] *P aeruginosa* strongly attacks the innate immune defense mechanism. It evades killing by promoting neutrophil apoptosis through production of pyocyanin and inhibits efferocytosis leading to secondary necrosis and tissue destruction.[53] *P aeruginosa* can also effectively escape immune attacks through biofilm production. Some strains of *S aureus* or *S pyogenes* can survive in neutrophils and cause neutrophil lysis with resultant release of viable bacteria, thus perpetuating the infectious process. In the case of *S aureus*, this resembles neutrophilic necroptosis where there is controlled leakage of cell contents through the plasma membrane. In addition, after ingestion of these bacteria, neutrophils express increased CD47 (known as the don't-eat-me signal), which interferes with efferocytosis.[52] *S aureus* and *S pyogenes* also produce plasma membrane pore-forming toxins that lead to neutrophil cytolysis.[52,54]

THE WOUND BIOBURDEN

Bioburden is defined as the number of viable microorganisms present on a surface or in a sample before terminal sterilization before human use. It is a term borrowed from the pharmaceutical and medical device industries. In the wound healing literature, it has come to represent the attributes of wound microbiology thought to be important in the development of wound infection, including microbial load, diversity, and microbial virulence.[55,56] How these wound bioburden attributes impair wound healing was discussed earlier.

Role of Wound Biofilm

To a large extent, the wound microbial load exists in a biofilm.[57] The prevalence of biofilms in wounds is thought to be 78% to 100%.[58] The presence of debris or implanted foreign bodies increases the likelihood of biofilm formation and chronic wound infection. Elek[59] showed that the presence of a silk suture reduced the required bacterial load for pustule formation from 7.5×10^6 to 10^2 organisms. It has also been shown that high inocula (10^8 CFU/mL) of *S aureus* in animal soft tissues do not lead to abscess formation. However, in the presence of a foreign body, 10^2 CFU/mL of *S aureus* caused an infection in 95% of the patients.[60] Foreign body presence significantly downregulates the phagocytosis and intracellular bactericidal effects of polymorphonuclear leukocytes.[61,62] As popularized by Bjarnsholt, there is growing evidence that bioburden and/or biofilm is a universal barrier to healing in all chronic wounds.[63–67] In the human microbiome, bacteria are generally present as aggregates. When embedded within the wound, these aggregates become immobile (sessile). Initially, this embedding is reversible and the innate immune response can remove the microbes (eg, in acute, well-vascularized wounds). However, in wounds where ischemia, tissue necrosis, or immunosuppression from disease or medication exist, and the microbes are not quickly cleared, a biofilm rapidly develops.[68,69] The sessile bacterial aggregate begins to secrete a matrix composed of polysaccharides, proteins, glycolipids, and bacterial DNA.[70–72] Within this biofilm environment, diverse bacteria share defense mechanisms and virulence factors that reduce antimicrobial and biocide effectiveness and augment survival of the aggregate microbial flora.[73–85] Although both are affected, reduced biofilm penetration by biocides seems more important than for antibiotics.[63,86–91] Biofilm bacteria produce PAMPs (eg, bacterial DNA and cell wall LPS), which induce polymorphonuclear leukocyte chemotaxis and increased production of proinflammatory cytokines, creating a persistent inflammatory state.[92,93] In addition, biofilm populated by P aeruginosa is a potent inducer of the M1 hyperinflammatory macrophage phenotype, and controls biofilm cellular quorum sensing to produce rhamnolipid, which leads to rapid necrosis (not apoptosis) of neutrophils.[94,95] Rapid lysis of neutrophils would be expected to release elastase, MMP, and proinflammatory cytokines, which perpetuate the inflammatory state.[96] This persistent inflammatory state stalls tissue repair (discussed earlier).

Role of Hypoxia

When local wound oxygen tension is measured, healing tissue is consistently hypoxic.[97,98] This tissue hypoxia has been shown to be important in facilitating many aspects of repair.[99–102] However, hypoxia has also been shown to facilitate bacterial infection. The seminal work of Hunt and colleagues,[103] in animals bearing wound cages, inoculated with P aeruginosa, and treated with oxygen atmospheres of 12%, 21%, and 45%, the residual colony counts and established infections were highest in the anoxic and lowest in the hyperoxic groups. Subsequent studies showed that hyperoxia could block E coli–induced tissue necrosis.[104] Low human wound transcutaneous oximetry levels are associated with wound infection as defined by quantitative bacterial culture.[105] Ischemia from arterial insufficiency substantially contributes to the wound bioburden.[106] The combination of infection and peripheral arterial disease has been shown to triple the likelihood of failed wound healing.[107] Infection is frequently the instigating event that leads to amputation in the threatened ischemic limb.[107–110]

The oxygen tension decreases from the periphery to the center of the wound bed.[111] Arterial insufficiency and increased oxygen consumption by neutrophils and microorganisms in wound biofilm exacerbate the central wound hypoxia.[101,102,112] Hypoxia has been shown to inhibit neutrophil apoptosis.[113]

Definition of Infection

Infectious disease specialists maintain that wounds are universally colonized with microbes because of loss of the protection of intact skin. Colonization is commonly defined as the presence of microorganisms in or on a host, with growth and multiplication, but without tissue invasion or cellular injury.[114] In their opinion, the wound is not infected until there are classic clinical findings of inflammation and/or purulent drainage present.[115–118]

Compared with colonization, infection a priori implies tissue invasion and cellular injury. The controversy therefore lies in the definition of infection and whether the classic clinical signs of inflammation, as described by Aulus Cornelius Celsus (45 AD), accurately describe the occurrence of tissue invasion and cellular injury that impairs tissue repair, particularly within the context of chronic infection. Celsus described the signs and symptoms of inflammation: rubor et tumor cum calore et dolore (redness and swelling with heat and pain). The fifth cardinal sign, functio laesa (disturbance of function), was added by Rudolph Virchow in 1858.[119] The four cardinal signs of Celsus only apply to acute inflammation accompanying wounds and infections, and functio laesa is the only universal sign that accompanies all inflammatory processes and characterizes chronic inflammation.[120]

Although inflammation stimulated by microbial infection and tissue damage is a manifestation of the innate immune response (discussed earlier), inflammation is not a synonym for infection. The clinical signs of inflammation primarily describe the body's immunoneurovascular response regardless of its cause, and the molecules and cells associated with inflammation are activated or expressed in high concentration in many conditions absent of tissue injury or infection.[121] Therefore, the classic clinical signs/symptoms of inflammation do not necessarily denote infection. The Infectious Disease Society of America (IDSA) defines infection as the presence of at least two of the following items: local swelling or induration, erythema, local tenderness or pain, local warmth, purulent discharge (thick, opaque to white, or sanguineous secretion); namely, the classic clinical signs of inflammation plus purulent drainage.[118] The identification of infection depends on the criteria used, and attempts to define infection purely by clinical signs and symptoms have been problematic. Leaper and colleagues,[122] in an assessment of the validity and reliability of the definition and measurement of surgical wound infection used in prospective studies, noted 41 different definitions of surgical wound infection. The presence of pus and the US Centers for Disease Control and Prevention (CDC) 1992 guidelines were the most frequently used. However, little has changed to date and none of these definitions have been validated.[122] Accordingly, the CDC/National Healthcare Safety Network does not define purulent drainage because there is no standard, clinically agreed-on definition.[123] As Leaper and colleagues[122] state, "It should be remembered that the 1992 CDC [guideline] definition now widely used in the UK and USA, has not been validated ... There is no single, objective gold standard test for surgical wound infection, and diagnosis is based variably on the presence and severity of a number of properties. Furthermore, judgement of wound status is highly subjective and at risk of intra- and inter-observer variation."[122] These definitions are for surgical wound infections, which, for the most part, start with incisions made in a sterile field. The problem becomes even more complicated when trying to define infection in diabetic and other chronic nonhealing wounds. O'Meara and colleagues[124] stated that, "We have not been able to identify the optimal methods of diagnosing infection in foot ulceration in diabetes. We know neither how to identify infection reliably by clinical assessment, nor which patients need formal diagnostic testing for infection ...." Nelson and colleagues[125] observed that, "The available evidence is too weak to be able to draw reliable implications for practice. This means that, in terms of diagnosis, infection in DFUs [diabetic foot ulcers] cannot be reliably identified using clinical assessment." Furthermore, no doubt contributing to these findings, in chronically infected wounds of patients with limb ischemia, peripheral neuropathy, or immunosuppression, the classic signs of inflammation may be absent[105,126]; and 50% of patients with a limb-threatening infection do not manifest systemic signs or symptoms.[127]

This point began to be addressed by the seminal work of Cutting and Harding[128] who, noting that the criteria used to identify surgical site infection were the finding of pus, or pus with inflammation,[128,129] echoed the view of Lawrence[130] "that the presence of pathogens in wounds not exhibiting visual evidence of infection cannot be ignored." Believing that traditional definitions of wound infection may be too narrow, they proposed additional criteria for the identification of wound infection that include: delayed healing; wound discoloration; friable; easily bleeding granulation tissue; unexpected pain and/or tenderness; pocketing at base of wound; bridging at base of wound; abnormal odor; and wound breakdown.[128] Because repair is the normal functional consequence of tissue injury, absence of repair indicates loss of function (functio laesa). Therefore, it seems reasonable that microbial interference with tissue repair should be included in the diagnosis of (particularly chronic) wound infection. Thus, these additions largely provided functio laesa elements of chronic nonhealing wounds to the infectious disease specialist's diagnosis of wound infection.

Validation of Definitions of Infection

The IDSA guidelines have been used as a method to stratify the infection component in studies examining outcomes of DFUs.[109,131] An additional study indirectly addressed the correlation between mild and no infection with blood levels of C-reactive protein.[132] However, there has been no validation of the 2012 IDSA guidelines with wound quantitative bacterial cultures. In a study specifically evaluating the IDSA diagnostic criteria for diabetic foot infections, Gardner and colleagues[105,131] carefully standardized the clinical assessment of these criteria and examined their association with bacterial load evaluated by quantitative bacterial cultures. They found the IDSA criteria for infection were not a valid predictor of bacterial load.[133] Similarly, in a comparable study in patients with chronic wounds of various origins, Gardner and colleagues[105] examined the association of the IDSA criteria and the additional criteria described by Cutting and Harding[128] with quantitative wound bacterial load. The investigators found that, in infected chronic wounds, the signs proposed by Cutting and Harding[128] were valid and seen more frequently than the IDSA criteria. They concluded that these signs seem to be the more valid indicators of chronic wound infection than the signs of classic inflammation, and it was suggested that meticulous attention be directed toward wounds with increasing wound pain, friable granulation tissue, foul odor, and wound breakdown because the data support their validity in predicting infection. The sensitivity of increasing wound pain and wound breakdown was 100%, indicating that, when present, the wound could be regarded as infected.[105] However, evidence is currently lacking to identify the optimal method to diagnose infection. The universal dependence on the classic signs of inflammation and/or pus does not seem warranted. For chronic wounds, increasing wound pain and wound breakdown seem promising adjuncts to the diagnosis, but reliance on clinical signs/symptoms alone is clearly not enough to diagnose infection. However, the extensive literature on the relationship between quantitative microbial cultures and wound and tissue closure outcomes is clearly persuasive (discussed earlier).

A Strategy for Deciding When Bacteria Are Interfering with Tissue Repair

As mentioned earlier, the attributes of wound microbiology thought important in the development of wound infection include not only microbial load but diversity and microbial virulence.[55,134] Quantification of each of these attributes and their relationship to wound outcomes seems to better approach a clear definition of infection. Although standard quantitative cultures begin to describe microbial load and diversity, the technique is laborious, dependent on sampling technique, dramatically underestimates the microbial load and diversity, and does not address virulence. Culture-based techniques select for those microorganisms that grow well under the typical nutritional and physiologic conditions used in standard diagnostic laboratories. Advances in molecular microbiological techniques to identify and quantify microorganisms have better informed clinicians' view of the wound microbiome. Current 16S ribosomal RNA gene sequencing allows characterization and quantification of the microbiome based on all three of the attributes mentioned earlier: microbial load, microbial diversity, and virulence.[134] Although these methods are becoming increasingly accessible and less expensive, they are clearly not ubiquitous. However, they seem to be critically important adjuncts in the ultimate definition of infection.

While waiting for these exciting developments, the current state of the art is that most tissue repair practitioners have only semiquantitative wound cultures available in their local armamentariums. Many clinical laboratories identify common microorganisms and report an indication of amount of growth (eg, 1+, 2+, 3+, 4+; or scant, light, moderate, numerous growth). This semiquantitative technique is based on dilutions of the bacterial load in sequential quadrants of the culture plate, and it roughly translates to less than 10^4, 10^4 to 10^5, 10^5 to 10^7, and greater than 10^7 CFU/g, respectively, for the gradations listed earlier.[135–137] With proper sampling techniques (ideally, sterilely obtained biopsy), use of these semiquantitative techniques, an understanding of the clinical signs and symptoms of chronic wound infection as defined by Cutting and Harding,[128] and with particular attention to the virulence of *Streptococcus*, *Pseudomonas*, and *S aureus* species, current practitioners can approach a rational definition of when the bacterial load is likely affecting tissue repair.

TREATMENT OF THE WOUND BIOBURDEN

Mature wound biofilms (chronic nonhealing wounds) require aggressive treatment composed of sharp wound debridement and adjunctive use of antimicrobial and other antibiofilm compounds. Frequent debridement with physical removal of microbial aggregates is thought to provide a brief (24–48 hours) opportunity during which the wound bacteria are most susceptible to antimicrobials.[63] The use of topical antimicrobials after debridement may help to prevent biofilm reformation or aid active killing of microbial cells where residual biofilm exists, without development of antibiotic resistance.[138]

Antibiotic Therapy

There is an established controversy regarding the use of antibiotics, both systemic and topical, for wounds. The debate exists between infectious disease specialists focused on antibiotic stewardship and wound healing specialists focused on tissue repair; these are clinically important foci that should not be mutually exclusive.

Tissue repair specialists might well ask a question: if, as this article shows, there are clear data to support the interference of bacteria with wound healing; the mechanism for that interference is now better understood; reducing the bacterial load allows tissue repair to proceed; and antimicrobials, including antibiotics, are critical to that reduction, why then is there a controversy over the use of antibiotics to reduce the bacterial burden?

Infectious disease specialists contend that the wound is not infected until there are classic clinical findings of inflammation and/or purulent drainage present. Accordingly, they contend, antibiotics should be reserved for infected wounds, and clinically uninfected wounds should not even be cultured.[115–118] They assert that antibiotics are needed to treat infections, not heal wounds.[117] Furthermore, infectious disease specialists decry the use of topical antibiotics in wound care and contend that topical antiseptics should be used.[115,116,118] The putative rationale for avoiding topical antibiotics is to avoid development of antibiotic resistance. However, this rationale seems to be based on opinion, because data for the occurrence of antibiotic resistance with topical antibiotics are lacking.[137–140] In addition, studies evaluating the toxicity of antibiotics and antiseptics at comparable antimicrobial concentrations clearly show the toxicity of antiseptics to wound cells is far greater than that of antibiotics.[141–149]

The wound specialists contend that the extensive data on impaired wound healing with microbial loads greater than or equal to 10^4 CFU/g show a threshold that requires antimicrobial intervention. They further contend that the infection definition adopted by the infectious disease specialists has not been validated as representative of bacterial load, thus clinging to this definition for recommending or discontinuing antibiotic use is tenuous. Additionally, they further contend that both systemic and topical antimicrobial agents have been a mainstay of wound care for more than 3600 years. From the Edwin Smith Papyrus of 1600 BC historically successful wound care was topical and involved agents that were antimicrobial.[150] The first antibiotics (sulfonamide and penicillin) saw extensive life-saving and limb-saving topical use in WWII battle wounds. Most modern wound dressings contain antimicrobial agents and recent meta-analyses support the use of an antimicrobial dressing instead of a nonantimicrobial dressing in increasing the number of diabetic foot ulcers healed over a medium-term follow-up period.[151]

Apropos of the earlier discussion, and as a vision of the future of wound care, Dowd and colleagues[138] evaluated molecular identification of the host and wound bioburden, frequent sharp debridement, use of antibiofilm wound dressings, and comprehensive standard care (revascularization, nutritional support, offloading, compression therapy, and management of comorbidities) in 1378 patients with wounds of various types. There were three cohorts: standard-of-care prescribed systemic antibiotics using empiric and traditional culture–based techniques, a second cohort that was prescribed an improved selection of systemic antibiotics based on molecular diagnostics, and a third cohort that received personalized topical therapeutics including topical antibiotics based on the results of molecular diagnostics. During the 7-month follow-up, 48.5% of the standard-of-care group healed completely, 62.4% of the second cohort with systemic antibiotics based on molecular diagnostics healed completely, and the cohort that received personalized topical antibiotics based on the results of molecular microbial identification had a 90.4% completed healing rate. Systemic antibiotic use was 29.4%, 50.7%, and 5.5% respectively. The patients receiving this tailored topical antibiotic therapy had a 200% better chance of healing at any given time point compared with cohorts receiving the same care without topical antibiotics.[138]

This review of the literature concerning bacteria, antibiotics and tissue repair shows there are extensive data supporting microbial interference with wound healing once bacterial burden exceeds 10^4 CFU per unit of measure. The mechanism of bacterial interference lies largely in prolonging the inflammatory phase of tissue repair. Reducing the microbial bioburden allows tissue repair to continue. Systemic and topical antimicrobials appear critical to reducing the bioburden and facilitating repair. The current controversy over the use of antimicrobials in patients with chronically infected wounds, in particular, revolves around the definition of infection. The reliance on classic clinical signs of inflammation to support antimicrobial use in these patients is tenuous due to the lack of correlation of these signs with the microbial burden known to impair tissue repair.

DISCLOSURE

The author has nothing to disclose.

REFERENCES

1. Nussbaum SR, Carter MJ, Fife CE, et al. An economic evaluation of the impact, cost, and medicare m policy implications of chronic nonhealing wounds. Value Health 2018;21:27–32.
2. Sen CK. Human wounds and its burden: an updated compendium of estimates. Adv Wound Care 2019;8(No. 2):39–48.
3. Breasted JH. Edwin Smith Surgical Papyrus. In: Facsimile and Hieroglyphic Transliteration with Translation and Commentary, 2 vols. Chicago: University of Chicago Oriental Institute Publications; 1930.
4. Hippocrates G, Coxe JR. The writings of Hippocrates and Galen. Philadelphia: Lyndsay and Blackiston; 1846.
5. Freiburg JA. The mythos of laudable pus along with an explanation for its origin. J Community Hosp Intern Med Perspect 2017;7(3):196–8.

6. Alexander JW. The contributions of infection control to a century of surgical progress. Ann Surg 1985;201:423–8.
7. Phillips LG, Heggers JP, Robson MC. History of quantitative bacteriology. In: Quantitative bacteriology: its role in the armamentarium of the surgeon. Boca Raton (FL): CRC Press; 1991. p. 9–14.
8. Tarmuzzer RW, Schultz GS. Biochemical analysis of acute and chronic wound environments. Wound Repair Regen 1996;4:321–5.
9. Thompson PD. Immunology, microbiology, and the recalcitrant wound. Ostomy Wound Manage 2000;46(suppl 1A):77S–82S.
10. Carrell A, Hartmann A. Cicatrization of wounds : I. the relation between the size of a wound and the rate of its cicatrization. J Exp Med 1916;24(5):429–50.
11. Hepburn HH. Delayed primary suture of wounds. Br Med J 1919;1(3033):181–3.
12. Altemeier WA. The bacteriology of war wounds. A collective review. Int Abstr Surg 1942;75:518.
13. Robson MC, Shaw RC, Heggers JP. The reclosure of postoperative incisionalabscesses based on bacterial quantification of the wound. Ann Surg 1970;171(2):279–82.
14. Howe CW. The early closure of constantly contaminated infected wounds with the aid of urethane-penicillin mixtures. Surg Gynecol Obstet 1948;87(4):425–34.
15. Liedburg NCF, Reiss E, Artz CP. The effect of bacteria on the take of split thickness skin grafts in rabbits. Ann Surg 1955;142:92.
16. Bendy RH Jr, Nuccio PA, Wolfe E, et al. Relationship of quantitative wound bacterial counts to healing of decubiti: effect of topical gentamicin. Antimicrob Agents Chemother 1964;10:147–55.
17. Krizek TJ, Robson MC, Kho E, et al. Bacterial growth and skin graft survival. Surg Forum 1967;18:518.
18. Robson MC, Lea CE, Dalton JB, et al. Quantitative bacteriology and delayed closure. Surg Forum 1968;19:501.
19. Robson MC, Heggers JP. Delayed wound closures based on bacterial counts. J Surg Oncol 1970;2(4):379–83.
20. Murphy MD, Robson MC, Heggers JP, et al. The effect of microbial contamination on musculocutaneous and random flaps. J Surg Res 1986;41(1):75–80.
21. Breidenbach WC, Trager S. Quantitative culture technique and infection in complex wounds of the extremities closed with free flaps. Plast Reconstr Surg 1995;95:860.
22. Majewski W, Cybulski Z, Napierala M, et al. The value of quantitative bacteriological investigations in the monitoring of treatment of ischaemic ulcerations of lower legs. Int Angiology 1995 Dec;14(4):381–4.
23. Høgsberg T, Bjahrnsholt T, Thomsen JS, et al. Success rate of split thickness skin grafting of chronic venous leg ulcers depends on the presence of Pseudomonas aeruginosa: a retrospective study. PLoS One 2011;6(5):1–6, e20492.
24. Xu L, McLennan SV, Lo L, et al. Bacterial load predicts healing rate in neuropathic diabetic foot ulcers. Diabetes Care 2007;30(2):378–80.
25. Lookingbill DP, Miller SH, Knowles RC. Bacteriology of chronic leg ulcers. Arch Dermatol 1978;114(12):1765–8.
26. Daltrey DC, Rhodes B, Chattwood JG. Investigation into the microbial flora of healing and non-healing decubitus ulcers. J Clin Pathol 1981;34:701–5.
27. Goldberg SR, Diegelmann RF. Wound healing primer. Surgical Clinics of North America 2010;90(6):1133–46.
28. Landén NX, Li D, Ståhle M. Transition from inflammation to proliferation: a critical step during wound healing. Cell Mol Life Sci 2016;73(20):3861–85.

29. Ellis S, Lin EJ, Tartar D. Immunology of wound healing. Curr Dermatol Rep 2018; 7(4):350–8.

30. Kawasaki T, Kawai T. Toll-like receptor signaling pathways. Front Immunol 2014; 5(461):1–8.

31. Kobayashi SD, Malachowa N, DeLeo FR. Influence of microbes on neutrophil life and death. Front Cell Infect Microbiol 2017;7:159.

32. Nauseef WM, Borregaard N. Neutrophils at work. Nat Immunol 2014;15:602–11.

33. Kobayashi SD, Braughton KR, Whitney AR, et al. Bacterial pathogens modulate an apoptosis differentiation program in human neutrophils. Proc Natl Acad Sci U S A 2003;100(19):10948–53.

34. Surewaard BG, de Haas CJ, Vervoort F, et al. Staphylococcal alpha-Phenol Soluble Modulins contribute to neutrophil lysis after phagocytosis. Cell Microbiol 2013;15(8):1427–37.

35. Kobayashi SD, Braughton KR, Palazzolo-Ballance AM, et al. Rapid Neutrophil Destruction following Phagocytosis of Staphylococcus aureus. J Innate Immun 2010;2:560–75.

36. Savill J, Haslett C. Granulocyte clearance by apoptosis in the resolution of inflammation. Cell Biol 1995;6:385–93.

37. Meszaros AJ, Reichner JS, Albina JE. Macrophage-induced neutrophil apoptosis. J Immunol 2000;165(1):435.

38. Daley JM, Reichner JS, Mahoney EJ, et al. Modulation of macrophage phenotype by soluble product(s) released from neutrophils. J Immunol 2005;174(4): 2265.

39. Khanna S, Biswas S, Shang Y, et al. Macrophage dysfunction impairs resolution of inflammation in the wounds of diabetic mice. PLoS One 2010;5(3):e9539.

40. Meszaros AJ, Reichner JS, Albina JE. Macrophage phagocytosis of wound neutrophils. J Leukoc Biol 1999;65(1):35–42.

41. Savill JS, Wyllie AH, Henson JE, et al. Macrophage phagocytosis of aging neutrophils in inflammation. Programmed cell death in the neutrophil leads to its recognition by macrophages. J Clin Invest 1989;83(3):865.

42. Fadok VA, Bratton DL, Konowal A, et al. Macrophages that have ingested apoptotic cells in vitro inhibit proinflammatory cytokine production through autocrine/paracrine mechanisms involving TGF-beta, PGE2, and PAF. J Clin Invest 1998;10(4):890.

43. Ferrante CJ, Leibovich SJ. Regulation of macrophage polarization and wound healing. Adv Wound Care 2012;1(1):10–6.

44. Krzyszczyk P, Schloss R, Palmer A, et al. The role of macrophages in acute and chronic wound healing and interventions to promote pro-wound healing phenotypes. Front Physiol 2018;9:419.

45. Hesketh M, Sahin KB, West ZE, et al. Macrophage phenotypes regulate scar formation and chronic wound healing. Int J Mol Sci 2017;18(7):1545.

46. Mills CD. Anatomy of a discovery: M1 and M2 macrophages. Front Immunol 2015;6:212.

47. Daley JM, Brancato SK, Thomay AA, et al. The phenotype of murine wound macrophages. J Leukoc Biol 2010;87:59–67.

48. Shook B, Xiao E, Kumamoto Y, et al. CD301b+ macrophages are essential for effective skin wound healing. J Invest Dermatol 2016;136:1885–91.

49. Zhao R, Liang H, Clarke E, et al. Inflammation in chronic wounds. Int J Mol Sci 2016;17(12):2085.

50. Sindrilaru A, Peters T, Wieschalka S, et al. An unrestrained proinflammatory M1 macrophage population induced by iron impairs wound healing in humans and mice. J Clin Invest 2011;121(3):985–97.
51. Loots MA, Lamme EN, Zeegelaar J, et al. Differences in cellular infiltrate and extracellular matrix of chronic diabetic and venous ulcers versus acute wounds. J Invest Dermatol 1998;111:850–7.
52. Kobayashi SD, Malachowa N, DeLeo FR. Neutrophils and Bacterial Immune Evasion. J Innate Immun 2018;10:432–41.
53. Fox S, Leitch AE, Duffin R, et al. Neutrophil apoptosis: relevance to the innate immune response and inflammatory disease. J Innate Immun 2010;2:216–27.
54. Brito C. Mechanisms protecting host cells against bacterial pore-forming toxins. Cell Mol Life Sci 2019;76:1319–39.
55. Gardner SE, Frantz RA. Wound bioburden and infection -related complications in diabetic foot ulcers. Bio Res Nurs 2008;10(1):44–53.
56. Dow G. Infection in chronic wounds. In: Krasner D, Rodeheaver G, Sibbald RG, editors. Chronic wound care: a clinical source book for healthcare professionals. Wayne (PA): HMP Communications; 2001. p. 343–56.
57. Percival SL, Hill KE, Williams DW, et al. Biofilms in wounds. Wound Repair Regen 2012;20:647–57.
58. Malone M, Bjarnsholt T, McBain AJ, et al. The prevalence of biofilms in chronic wounds: a systematic review and meta-analysis of published data. J Wound Care 2017;26(1):20–5.
59. Elek SD. Experimental staphylococcal infections in the skin of man. Ann N Y Acad Sci 1956;65:85.
60. Zimmerli W, Waldvogel FA, Vaudaux P, et al. Pathogenesis of foreign body infection: description and characteristics of an animal model. J Infect Dis 1982; 146(4):487–97.
61. Zimmerli W, Lew PD, Waldvogel FA. Pathogenesis of foreign body infection. Evidence for a local granulocyte defect. J Clin Invest 1984;73(4):1191–200.
62. Wu H, Moser C, Wang H, et al. Strategies for combating bacterial biofilm infections. Int J Oral Sci 2015;7:1–7.
63. Wolcott RD, Rumbaugh KP, James G, et al. Biofilm maturity studies indicate sharp debridement opens a time-dependent therapeutic window. J Wound Care 2010;19(8):320–8.
64. Wolcott RD, Rhoads DD, Dowd SE. Biofilms and chronic wound inflammation. J Wound Care 2008;17(8):333–41.
65. Wolcott RD, Rhoads DD, Bennett ME, et al. Chronic wounds and the medical biofilm paradigm. J Wound Care 2010;19(2):45–55.
66. Wolcott RD, Cox SB, Dowd SE. Healing and healing rates of chronic wounds in the age of molecular pathogen diagnostics. J Wound Care 2010;19(7):272–81.
67. Bjarnsholt T, Kirketerp-Møller K, Jensen PØ, et al. Why chronic wounds will not heal: a novel hypothesis. Wound Repair Regen 2008;16:2–10.
68. Bjarnsholt T, Eberlein T, Malone M, et al. Management of wound biofilm Made Easy. London. Wounds Int 2017;8(2):1–6.
69. James GA, Zhao AG, Usui M, et al. Microsensor and transcriptomic signatures of oxygen depletion in biofilms associated with chronic wounds. Wound Repair Regen 2016;24(2):373–83.
70. Flemming HC, Neu TR, Wozniak DJ. The EPS matrix: the "house of biofilm cells". J Bacteriol 2007;189(22):7945–7.
71. Sutherland I. Biofilm exopolysaccharides: a strong and sticky framework. Microbiology 2001;147(1):3–9.

72. Hall-Stoodley L, Stoodley P. Evolving concepts in biofilm infections. Cell Microbiol 2009;11(7):1034–43.

73. Donlan RM, Costerton JW. Biofilms: survival mechanisms of clinically relevant microorganisms. Clin Microbiol Rev 2002;15(2):67–93.

74. Xavier JB, Foster KR. Cooperation and conflict in microbial biofilms. Proc Natl Acad Sci U S A 2007;104(3):876–81.

75. Hibbing ME, Fuqua C, Parsek MR, et al. Bacterial competition: surviving and thriving in the microbial jungle. Nat Rev Microbiol 2010;8(1):15–25.

76. Harrison-Balestra C, Cazzaniga AL, Davis SC, et al. A wound-isolated Pseudomonas aeruginosa grows a biofilm in vitro within 10 hours and is visualized by light microscopy. Dermatol Surg 2003;29(6):631–5.

77. Leid JG, Willson CJ, Shirtliff ME, et al. The exopolysaccharide alginate protects Pseudomonas aeruginosa biofilm bacteria from IFN-gamma-mediated macrophage killing. J Immunol 2005;175(11):7512–8.

78. Ren D, Bedzyk LA, Thomas SM, et al. Gene expression in Escherichia coli biofilms. Appl Microbiol Biotechnol 2004;64(4):515–24.

79. Cho KH, Caparon MG. Patterns of virulence gene expression differ between biofilm and tissue communities of Streptococcus pyogenes. Mol Microbiol 2005; 57(6):1545–56.

80. Werner E, Roe F, Bugnicourt A, et al. Stratified growth in Pseudomonas aeruginosa biofilms. Appl Environ Microbiol 2004;70(10):6188–96.

81. Rani SA, Pitts B, Beyenal H, et al. Spatial patterns of DNA replication, protein synthesis, and oxygen concentration within bacterial biofilms reveal diverse physiological states. J Bacteriol 2007;189(11):4223–33.

82. Sauer K, Camper AK, Ehrlich GD, et al. Pseudomonas aeruginosa displays multiple phenotypes during development as a biofilm. J Bacteriol 2002;184:1140.

83. Fux CA, Costerton JW, Stewart PS, et al. Survival strategies of infectious biofilms. Trends Microbiol 2005;13(1):34–40.

84. Wolcott RD, Gontcharova V, Sun Y, et al. Evaluation of the bacterial diversity among and within individual venous leg ulcers using bacterial tag-encoded FLX and titanium amplicon pyrosequencing and metagenomic approaches. BMC Microbiol 2009;9:226.

85. Fey PD. Modality of bacterial growth presents unique targets: how do we treat biofilm-mediated infections? Curr Opin Microbiol 2010;13:610–5.

86. Stewart PS, Costerton JW. Antibiotic resistance of bacteria in biofilms. Lancet 2001;358(9276):135–8.

87. Stewart PS. Mechanisms of antibiotic resistance in bacterial biofilms. Int J Med Microbiol 2002;292(2):107–13.

88. Rose H, Baldwin A, Dowson CG, et al. Biocide susceptibility of the Burkholderia cepacia complex. J Antimicrob Chemother 2009;63(3):502–10.

89. Costerton JW, Stewart PS. Battling biofilms. Sci Am 2001;285(1):74–81.

90. Stewart PS, Rayner J, Roe F, et al. Biofilm penetration and disinfection efficacy of alkaline hypochlorite and chlorosulfamates. J Appl Microbiol 2001;91(3): 525–32.

91. Stewart PS, Davison WM, Steenbergen JN. Daptomycin rapidly penetrates a Staphylococcus epidermidis biofilm. Antimicrob Agents Chemother 2009; 53(8):3505–7.

92. Bayles KW. The biological role of death and lysis in biofilm development. Nat Rev Microbiol 2007;5:721–6.

93. Zhao G, Usui ML, Underwood RA, et al. Time course study of delayed wound healing in a biofilm-challenged diabetic mouse model. Wound Repair Regen 2012;20:342–52.
94. Ciszek-Lenda M, Strus M, Walczewska M, et al. Pseudomonas aeruginosa biofilm is a potent inducer of phagocyte hyperinflammation. Inflamm Res 2019;68: 397–413.
95. Jensen PØ, Bjarnsholt T, Phipps R, et al. Rapid necrotic killing of polymorphonuclear leukocytes is caused by quorum-sensing-controlled production of rhamnolipid by Pseudomonas aeruginosa. Microbiol 2007;153:1329–38.
96. Nwomeh BC, Yager DR, Cohen IK. Physiology of the chronic wound. Clin Plast Surg 1998;25:341–56.
97. Sheffield PJ. Tissue oxygen measurements. In: Davis JC, Hunt TK, editors. Problem wounds: the role of oxygen. New York: Elsevier; 1988. p. 17–52.
98. Silver IA. Wound healing and cellular microenvironment. London: European Research Office, United States Army; 1971.
99. Knighton DR, Silver IA, Hunt TK. Regulation of wound-healing angiogenesis—effect of oxygen gradients and inspired oxygen concentration. Surgery 1981; 90:262–70.
100. Hopf HW, Gibson JJ, Angeles AP, et al. Hyperoxia and angiogenesis. Wound Repair Regen 2005;13:558–64.
101. Tandara A, Mustoe T. Oxygen in wound healing—more than a nutrient. World J Surg 2004;28:294–300.
102. Bishop A. Role of Oxygen in wound healing. J Wound Care 2008;17(9):399–402.
103. Hunt TK, Linsey M, Grislis H, et al. The effect of differing ambient oxygen tensions on wound infection. Ann Surg 1975;181:35–9.
104. Knighton DR, Halliday B, Hunt TK. Oxygen as an antibiotic: the effect of inspired oxygen on infection. Arch Surg 1984;119(2):199–204.
105. Gardner SE, Frantz RA, Doebbeling BN. The validity of the clinical signs and symptoms used to identify localized chronic wound infection. Wound Repair Regen 2001;9:178–86.
106. Ahn ST, Mustoe TA. Effects of ischemia on ulcer wound healing: a new model in the rabbit ear. Ann Plast Surg 1990;24(1):17–23.
107. Prompers L, Schaper N, Apelqvist J, et al. Prediction of outcome in individuals with diabetic foot ulcers: focus on the differences between individuals with and without peripheral arterial disease. The EURODIALE Study. Diabetologia 2008; 51:747–55.
108. Mills JL, Conte MS, Armstrong DG, et al, on behalf of the Society for Vascular Surgery Lower Extremity Guidelines Committee. The Society for vascular surgery lower extremity threatened limb classification system: risk stratification based on wound, ischemia, and foot infection (WIfI). J Vasc Surg 2014;59(1): 220–34.e2.
109. Prompers L, Huijberts M, Apelqvist J, et al. High prevalence of ischaemia, infection and serious comorbidity in patients with diabetic foot disease in Europe. Baseline results from the Eurodiale study. Diabetologia 2007;50:18–25.
110. Brass EP, Anthony R, Dormandy J, et al. Parenteral therapy with lipo-ecraprost, a lipid-based formulation of a PGE1 analog, does not alter six-month outcomes in patients with critical leg ischemia. J Vasc Surg 2006;43:752–9.
111. Lundberg G, Walberg E, Swedenborg J, et al. Continuous assessment of local metabolism by microdialysis in critical limb ischemia. Eur J Vasc Endovasc Surg 2000;19:605–13.

112. Schaffer K, Taylor CT. The impact of hypoxia on bacterial infection. FEBS J 2015; 282:2260–6.

113. Walmsley SR, Print C, Farahi N, et al. Hypoxia-induced neutrophil survival is mediated by HIF-1alpha-dependent NF-kappaB activity. J Exp Med 2005; 201(1):105-115.

114. The Gale Group, Inc.; Gale Encyclopedia of Medicine. 2008.

115. IWGDF Guidelines on the prevention and management of diabetic foot disease. The International Working Group on the Diabetic Foot 2019. Available at: https://iwgdfguidelines.org/. Accessed June 16, 2020.

116. Lipsky BA, Dryden M, Gottrup F, et al. Antimicrobial stewardship in wound care: A Position Paper from the British Society for Antimicrobial Chemotherapy and European Wound Management Association. J Antimicrob Chemother 2016; 71(11):3026–35.

117. Abbas M, Uckay I, Lipsky BA. In diabetic foot infections antibiotics are to treat infection, not to heal wounds. Expert Opin Pharmacother 2015;16:821–32.

118. Lipsky BA, Berendt AR, Cornia PB, et al. 2012 infectious diseases society of america clinical practice guideline for the diagnosis and treatment of diabetic foot infections. Clin Infect Dis 2012;54(12):e132–73.

119. Majno G. The healing hand - man and wound in the ancient world. Cambridge (MA): Harvard University Press; 1975.

120. Medzhitov R. Inflammation 2010: New adventures of an old flame. Cell 2010; 140(6):19, 771–6.

121. Antonelli M, Kushner I. It's time to redefine inflammation. FASEB J 2017;31: 1787–91.

122. Leaper D, Tanner J, Kierna M. Surveillance of surgical site infection: more accurate definitions and intensive recording needed. J Hosp Infect 2001;49:99–108.

123. Available at: https://www.cdc.gov/nhsn/faqs/faq-ssi.html. Accessed June 16, 2020.

124. O'Meara S, Nelson EA, Golder S, et al, on behalf of the DASIDU Steering Group. Systematic review of methods to diagnose infection in foot ulcers in diabetes. Diabet Med 2006;23:341–7.

125. Nelson EA, O'Meara S, Craig D, et al. A series of systematic reviews to inform a decision analysis for sampling and treating infected diabetic foot ulcers (DA-SIDU). Health Technol Assess 2006;10(1):iii–iv, ix-x, 1-221.

126. Lavery LA, Armstrong DG, Murdoch DP, et al. Validation of the Infectious Diseases Society of America's diabetic foot infection classification system. Clin Infect Dis 2007;44(4):562–5.

127. Lipsky BA, Berendt AR, Deery HG, et al. Diagnosis and treatment of diabetic foot infections. Clin Infect Dis 2004;39:885–910.

128. Cutting KF, Harding KG. Criteria for identifying wound infection. J Wound Care 1994;3(4):198–201.

129. Meers PD, Ayliffe GAJ, Emmerson AM, et al. Report on the national survey of infection in hospitals, 1980. J Hosp Infect 1981;2(supplement):29–34.

130. Lawrence, J.C. The effect of bacteria and their products on the healing of skin wounds. In: Rue, Y. (ed.). A Biological Approach to the Wound Healing Process: A clinical update. (Proceedings of a symposium held at the Royal College of Physicians, London, June 5, 1987.) Andover: Medifax, 1987

131. Gardner SE, Frantz RA, Saltzman CL. Diabetes and inflammation in infected chronic wounds. Wounds 2005;17(8):203–5.

132. Jeandrot A, Richard JL, Combescure C, et al. Serum procalcitonin and C-reactive protein concentrations to distinguish mildly infected from non-infected diabetic foot ulcers: a pilot study. Diabetologia 2008;51(2):347–52.
133. Gardner SE, Hillis SL, Frantz RA. Clinical signs of infection in diabetic foot ulcers with high microbial load. Biol Res Nurs 2009;11(2):119–28.
134. Misic AM, Gardner SE, Grice EA. The wound microbiome: modern approaches to examining the role of microorganisms in impaired chronic wound healing. Adv Wound Care 2014;3(7):502–10.
135. Navarria L, Loda M, Bertolini A, et al. Validation of a new tool for a semi-quantitative bacterial growth with isolated colonies using a 4 quadrant streaking pattern on the WASP, European Society of Clinical Microbiology and Infectious Disease. 2015. Available at: https://www.escmid.org/escmid_publications/escmid_elibrary/?q=laura%20Navarria&tx_solr%5Bfilter%5D%5B0%5D=entry_type%253APoster%2Bpresentation. Accessed June 16, 2020.
136. Thomas PD. What is infection? Am J Surg 1994;167(1 A):7S–11S.
137. Vanaja R, Banu SG. Role of semiquantitative bacteriological culture in management of chronic wound infections. Indian J Microbiol Res 2018;5(3):398–403.
138. Dowd SE, Wolcott RD, Kennedy J, et al. Molecular diagnostics and personalised medicine in wound care: assessment of outcomes. J Wound Care 2011;20(5):232, 234–9.
139. Wall GM, Stroman DW, Roland PS, et al. Ciprofloxacin 0.3%/dexamethasone 0.1% sterile otic suspension for the topical treatment of ear infections: a review of the literature. Pediatr Infect Dis 2009;28(2):141–4.
140. Weber PC, Roland PS, Hannley M, et al. The development of antibiotic resistant organisms with the use of ototopical medications. Otolaryngology-Head and Neck Surgery 2004;130(35):589–94.
141. Teepe RG, Koebrugge EJ, Löwik CW, et al. Cytotoxic effects of topical antimicrobial and antiseptic agents on human keratinocytes in vitro. J Trauma 1993;35(1):8–19.
142. Tatnall FM, Leigh IM, Gibson JR. Assay of antiseptic agents in cell culture: conditions affecting cytotoxicity. J Hosp Infect 1991;17:287.
143. Damour O, Hua SZ, Lasne F, et al. Cytotoxicity evaluation of antiseptics and antibiotics on cultured human fibroblasts and keratinocytes. Burns 1992;18(6):479.
144. Brennan SS, Leaper DJ. The effect of antiseptics on the healing wound: a study using the rabbit ear chamber. Br J Surg 1985;72:780.
145. Lineaweaver W, Howard R, Soucy D, et al. Topical antimicrobial toxicity. Arch Surg 1985;120:267.
146. Welch H, Brewer CM. The toxicity-indices of some basic antiseptic substances. J Immunology 1942;43:25–30.
147. Müller G, Kramer A. Biocompatibility index of antiseptic agents by parallel assessment of antimicrobial activity and cellular cytotoxicity. J Antimicrob Chemother 2008;61:1281.
148. Marquardt C, Matuschek E, Bölke E, et al. Evaluation of the tissue toxicity of antiseptics by the hen's egg test on the chorioallantoic membrane (HETCAM). Eur J Med Res 2010;15:204.
149. McDonnell G, Russell AD. Antiseptics and disinfectants: activity, action, and resistance. Microbiol Rev 1999;12(1):147.
150. Caldwell MD. Topical wound therapy – an historic perspective. J Trauma 1990; 30(19):S116–22.
151. Dumville JC, Lipsky BA, Hoey C, et al. Topical antimicrobial agents for treating foot ulcers in people with diabetes. Cochrane Database Syst Rev 2017;(6):CD011038.

Defining the Role of Hyperbaric Oxygen Therapy as an Adjunct to Reconstructive Surgery

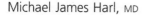

Michael James Harl, MD

KEYWORDS

- Hyperbaric oxygen • Reconstructive surgery • Crush injuries
- Compartment syndrome • Compromised flap • Reperfusion injury • Burn

KEY POINTS

- Hyperbaric oxygen therapy is a useful but underutilized adjunct to wound care and reconstructive surgery.
- Surgical and nonsurgical indications for hyperbaric oxygen therapy follow 2 general patterns of ischemia, which are the trichotomy of perfusion and ischemia-reperfusion.
- The final common pathway for surgical and nonsurgical hyperbaric oxygen therapy is leukocyte adhesion to endothelium and the subsequent lipid peroxidation, both of which are ameliorated by hyperbaric oxygen therapy.

It is an academic error, as well as a transgression of common decency, for any plastic surgeon to discuss this topic without first acknowledging the contributions of William A. Zamboni, MD, FACS. His contributions to this subject are extensive yet underappreciated. Despite this body of work, HBOT has been slow to be accepted by reconstructive and wound care surgeons alike.

There are some obvious barriers to this acceptance, such as limited access to hyperbaric chambers and staff, especially during off hours, when these conditions need emergent/urgent attention; lack of institutional enthusiasm, because these treatments consume valuable diagnosis-related group revenue; possible lack of insurance reimbursement based on local coverage determinants, when these treatments are extended to the outpatient period; and surgeon bias and the view that HBOT is a technology searching for a purpose.

This article addresses only the surgeon bias in hopes that achieving increased acceptance from the surgical community will create the momentum to overcome the other barriers.

Author note: No declarations or conflicts of interest.
Department of Plastic Surgery, Marshfield Clinic Health Care System, 611 North Saint Joseph Avenue, Marshfield, WI 54449, USA
E-mail address: harl.michael@marshfieldclinic.org

The article begins by reviewing conditions where there is uniform acceptance of the role of HBOT in their treatment and then demonstrates that these conditions have similar pathophysiologic derangements as conditions commonly encountered by the reconstructive and wound care surgeon. Each section concludes with a brief review of some of the experimental and clinical data showing the benefit of HBOT in the treatment of these conditions.

INDICATIONS
Universally Accepted Indications

Among the indications for hyperbaric oxygen therapy (HBOT), as determined by the Undersea and Hyperbaric Medical Society (UHMS),[1] the indications discussed seem universally accepted. This is in no way to imply a complete absence of controversy.

Carbon monoxide poisoning

Treatment of carbon monoxide poisoning traditionally has focused on reducing the hypoxic stress brought about by the elevated carboxyhemaglobin level. Carbon monoxide is known to cause cardiac injury, motor weakness, peripheral neuropathies, hearing loss, and Parkinson-like syndrome.[2] The negative sequalae that carbon monoxide poisoning shares with the reconstructive surgical indications are the adhesion of leukocytes to injured microvasculature and the resultant lipid peroxidation[2] (**Fig. 1**).

If there is a period of syncope or even a brief episode of hypotension during an episode of carbon monoxide poisoning, lipid peroxidation can be initiated. Carbon monoxide can enhance the rate of release of nitric oxide from both platelets and endothelial cells. The resultant nitric oxide–mediated changes are necessary for leukocyte adherence to cerebral microvasculature. Once the leukocytes are adherent to the endothelial cells, leukocyte activation occurs. This activation results in the release of reactive oxygen species (ROS) that convert xanthine dehydrogenase to xanthine oxidase, which is required for lipid peroxidation to ensue.[3] Thom and colleagues[3] note that the mechanism of cerebral injury associated with carbon monoxide poisoning is similar to postanoxic encephalopathy, which is a form of ischemic reperfusion injury.

HBOT has been shown to prevent brain oxidative injury in animals by inhibiting β2 integrin–mediated leukocyte adherence to endothelial cells[3,4] and that HBOT at 2.8 atmospheres absolute (ATAs) to 3 ATAs inhibits the function of β2 integrin in human polymorphonuclear cells.[3–5]

Decompression illness

One of the earliest recognized and most frequently touted uses for HBOT is in the treatment of decompression illness (DCI), or the bends. DCI describes a spectrum of injuries ranging from the purely cutaneous cutis marmorata to air gas emboli. The underlying mechanism for DCI is the formation of inert gas bubbles (typically nitrogen) in blood and tissues due to supersaturation of the gas,[6] which can occur with scuba diving or anytime an individual is breathing air at increased atmospheric pressures (eg, caisson disease) followed by rapid ascent to altitude.

Despite DCI being one of the first known uses for HBOT, the exact pathology in humans is not fully known. This is because study has been hampered by the lack of reproducible animal models.[7] The primary mechanism by which bubbles are thought to exert their deleterious effects is by mechanical occlusion of blood flow. HBOT improves the condition by simply decreasing bubble size by mechanical means combined with nitrogen washout. Divers with low bubble production, however, have been shown to develop symptoms of DCI, and divers with high bubble production

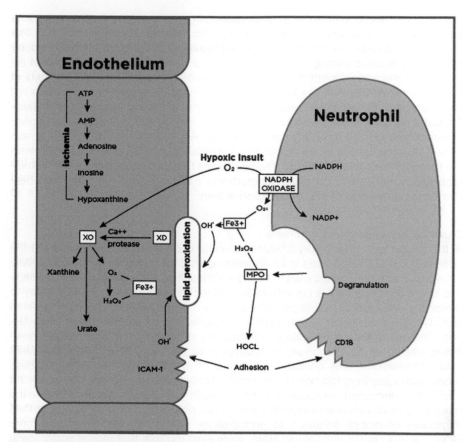

Fig. 1. Leukocyte adhesion to endothelium and the subsequent lipid peroxidation. AMP, adenosine monophosphate; HOCL, hypochlorous acid; MPO, myeloperoxidase; NADP, nicotinamide adenine dinucleotide phosphate; NADPH, the reduced form of NADP; XD, xanthine dehydrogenase; XO, Xanthine Oxidase.

do not necessarily develope DCI.[8] Interestingly, bubbles have been shown to cause platelet activation[9] and to affect leukocyte-endothelial cell interaction.[10] Therefore, it is likely that the beneficial effects of HBOT extend beyond simple bubble mechanics.

Madden and colleagues[11] hypothesize that "gas bubbles are not the causative agent in progression of DCI, but rather an exacerbating factor." It has been demonstrated that β2 integrin–mediated leukocyte adhesion is associated with neurologic deterioration after decompression stress in rats and that prophylactic HBOT can improve outcomes.[12] Even so-called silent bubbles have been shown to impair endothelial-dependent vasoactive responses and to increase neutrophil infiltration.[13] Zamboni and colleagues[14] have demonstrated that HBOT produced sharp reduction in the adherence of leukocytes in the venules of postischemic muscle and that, by blocking leukocyte action, the no-reflow phenomenon may be abated.

Conditions Encountered by Reconstructive and Wound Care Surgeons

It often is said that the answer to almost every question in reconstructive surgery is blood flow. This can be translated more specifically to mean oxygen delivery. Many of the problems encountered in reconstructive surgery, wound care, and medicine in general can be understood in terms of their specific aberration in oxygen delivery. The conditions that follow are those commonly encountered by reconstructive and wound care surgeons and are thought to benefit from the adjunctive use of HBOT. It is helpful to think of them as different manifestations of ischemia-reperfusion injury. Many of these conditions manifest the trichotomy of perfusion. That is to say that there will be an area with adequate perfusion, an area with no perfusion, and in-between these 2 areas a region of marginal perfusion. It is at this area of marginal perfusion, or penumbra, where HBOT exerts its greatest influence. Any injury state that has an element of ischemia-reperfusion or the trichotomy of perfusion (or both) likely will benefit from the timely administration of HBOT. The injury state that best exemplifies the ischemia-reperfusion model is crush injury/compartment syndrome, and the injury that best demonstrates the trichotomy of perfusion is burn.

Crush injury/compartment syndrome
At the cellular level, crush injury produces a vicious cycle of edema, hypoxia, and more edema. If this process occurs in an enclosed space, the microcirculation completely collapses and further contributes to the hypoxic insult until irreversible tissue damage has occurred. Eventually, a fasciotomy is required to restore blood flow. One way to arrest the progression of this process is to disrupt the vicious cycle early on with HBOT.[15] Once perfusion is temporarily interrupted, however, the endothelium becomes sensitized to the hypoxic insult, resulting in the activation of adhesion molecules, leading to the attachment of neutrophils to the endothelium and subsequent lipid peroxidation.[15] The deleterious cascade of events associated with ischemia-reperfusion injury from this point on resemble elements of carbon monoxide poisoning and DCI, as discussed previously, with ROS converting the dehydrogenase form to the oxidase form of xanthine oxidoreductase, which produces further ROS, which then stimulates neutrophil adhesion to endothelium, and which then produces more ROS.[16] In the normal physiologic state, there exist multiple free radical scavengers, such as superoxide dismutase, glutathione, and catalase. In ischemia-reperfusion injury, however, they are rapidly overwhelmed.[16]

HBOT has a unique, seemingly paradoxic, benefit in preventing compartment syndrome by reducing edema via vasoconstriction[17] while maintaining tissue oxygenation as a result of plasma hyperoxygenation.[18] Unfortunately, HBOT consultation rarely is obtained in the setting of impending compartment syndrome. Rather, if it is obtained, it is done after the compartment release, when threatened tissue loss is observed. HBOT potentially still is beneficial in this setting by mitigating the effects of ongoing ischemia-reperfusion injury by blocking the adhesion of neutrophils to the endothelium and stopping the release of ROS. Earlier use of HBOT, however, leads to a more significant reduction in tissue damage.[15]

Thermal burns
Classic teaching describes the burn wound as having 3 zones: a central zone of coagulation, surrounded by an area of stasis, which is surrounded by an area of erythema. At a tissue level, this represents an oxygen gradient. Most chronic wounds also have an oxygen gradient, and it has been shown that HBOT improves healing by increasing this gradient and stimulating neoangiogenesis.[19]

The zone of coagulation usually is not salvageable, and the zone of hyperemia almost always heals. So, any efforts to reduce the size of the burn and healing time typically focus on the zone of stasis (the penumbra); this is an attempt to prevent the conversion of this burn from a partial-thickness burn to a full-thickness burn. These 3 zones represent the trichotomy of perfusion seen with most thermal burns.

One of the main factors affecting hypoxia in the zone of stasis is edema, and a decrease in edema has been shown to decrease burn conversion from partial thickness to full thickness.[20] Edema is most evident in the burned tissues but also develops in distant, unburned tissue. It has been demonstrated that this edema generation is from increased capillary permeability and is the result of more than just thermal injury. Changes have been demonstrated in the distant microvasculature, including red cell aggregation, white cell adhesion to venular walls, platelet microthrombi, and complement activation.[21,22] Also, failure of the sodium pump as a result of reduced intracellular adenosine triphosphate (ATP) is felt to be a major factor in the swelling of endothelial cells and the resultant edema.[21] Lastly, it has been demonstrated that there is an element of ischemia-reperfusion injury in the burn with activation of neutrophils, production of xanthine oxidase, release of ROS, and the resultant lipid peroxidation.[22] Ward and Till[22] speculate that the burn activates complement, which in turn activates neutrophils, causing them to adhere to the endothelium of the interstitial capillaries of the lung, leading to some of the pulmonary complications associated with burn injuries.

The effects on burn injury that are shared with the other indications for HBOT are the reduction of edema while increasing oxygenation via vasoconstriction and plasma hyperoxygenation, increasing intracellular ATP and decreasing endothelial cell swelling, and blocking neutrophil adhesion to endothelium, which blocks the release of ROS, thus preventing lipid peroxidation.

Cianci and colleagues[23] have demonstrated numerous beneficial effects of HBOT in the burn patient, which likely extend well beyond just treating the cutaneous injury. Their 2013 article leaves little room to debate the benefits of HBOT, yet most burn patients never see the inside of a hyperbaric chamber. This likely is because most burn units lack access to hyperbaric centers that are capable of diving a critically injured burn patient.

Compromised flaps
All flaps by their nature experience some degree of ischemic insult and this typically occurs at the time of transfer or transposition. Flaps are broadly placed into 1 of 2 categories. They are either a free flap, which has its blood supply divided and is transferred to a new, remote location using microsurgery, or are categorized as pedicled flaps, which are left attached to their blood supply and transposed to a nearby location. The ischemic insult experienced by free flaps is dominated by the ischemia-reperfusion model, whereas the pedicled flaps more clearly demonstrate the trichotomy of flow. Both have been shown to benefit from HBOT.

Zamboni and Baynosa[24] states that "HBOT is neither necessary nor recommended for the support of normal, uncompromised grafts or flaps. However, in tissue compromised by irradiation or in cases where there is decreased perfusion or hypoxia, HBOT has been shown to be extremely useful in flap salvage. Hyperbaric therapy can help maximize the viability of the compromised tissue thereby reducing the need for re-grafting or repeat flap procedures."

Using a skeletal muscle microcirculatory model of ischemia-reperfusion injury, Zamboni and colleagues[25] demonstrated that HBOT reduces neutrophil endothelial adherence in venules and suggests that HBOT is affecting the neutrophil CD18 adhesion molecule. In support of this, using a superior epigastric-based transverse rectus abdominis myocutaneous flap ischemia-reperfusion model in rats, Hong and colleagues[26] demonstrated that HBOT decreases the expression of the adhesion molecule ICAM-1 on endothelial cells.

Clinical studies have shown improvement of ischemic flaps, especially if HBOT is initiated within 24 hours of the ischemic insult.[25,26] The key point is the recognition of the ischemic event before irreversible tissue damage has occurred. Intraoperative fluorescent angiography can demonstrate areas of poor perfusion and, in the author's experience, assuming mechanical causes have been excluded, then HBOT is

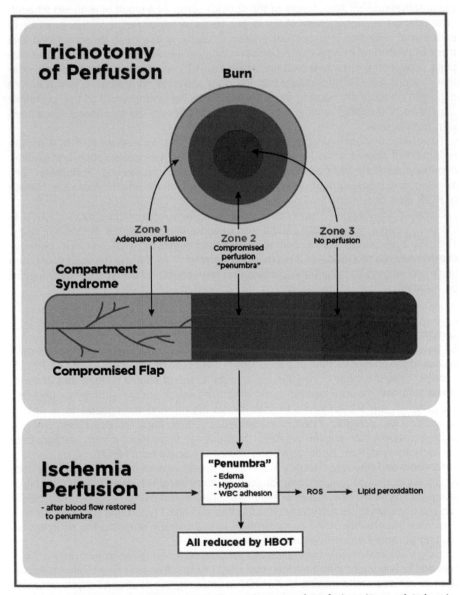

Fig. 2. The 2 patterns of ischemia. (*Top*) The trichotomy of perfusion. (*Bottom*) Ischemia-perfusion. WBC, white blood cell.

considered. Ideally, an intubated patient is taken directly from the operating room to the hyperbaric chamber for treatment. After the treatment, the patient would be taken to the intensive care unit for extubation and flap monitoring. At this time, logistical issues prevent this sequence from happening, so emphasis is made on the patient receiving the first treatment within 24 hours of surgery.

TREATMENT PROTOCOLS
Carbon Monoxide Poisoning

Two treatment protocols are listed by the UHMS. The first is the Weaver protocol, which consists of providing 3 ATAs of oxygen for 25 minutes, followed by a 5-minute air break, followed by another 3 ATAs of oxygen for 25 minutes, then a 5-minute air break, followed by chamber depressurization to 2 ATAs of oxygen for 30 minutes, 5-minute air break, 2 ATAs of oxygen for 30 minutes, and then depressurizing to barometric pressure.[2]

The Thom protocol is 2.8 ATAs of oxygen for 30 minutes, followed by 2 ATAs of oxygen for 90 minutes.[2] With either treatment protocol, patients should have electrocardiogram, serial troponins, and frequent neurologic examinations. Multiple treatments frequently are required, and cognitive and neurologic sequalae can occur weeks after the initial insult.

Decompression Illness

The treatment protocols for DCI are vast and vary depending on the inhaled gas and the depth/pressure at which the gas is inspired. The interested reader is referred to the US Navy and National Oceanic and Atmospheric Administration dive tables as well as current recommendations from the UHMS.

Crush Injuries and Compartment Syndromes

Strauss[15] recommends that HBOT be considered in patients with Gustilo types IIIB and IIIC fractures and in lesser Gustilo types in impaired hosts. The recommended treatment is 2 ATAs to 2.4 ATAs for 90 minutes for 2 treatments per day, or 120 minutes once a day.[15] HBOT is recommended after fasciotomy if significant residual problems remain. These include ischemic muscle, threatened flaps, residual neuropathy, massive edema, and ischemic time greater than 6 hours. HBOT protocols after fasciotomy are the same as for crush injuries.[15]

Thermal Burns

It is recommended that treatment with HBOT begin as early as possible, attempting 3 treatments within the first 24 hours and twice daily thereafter. This should be 100% oxygen at 2 ATAs to 2.4 ATAs for 90 minutes.[23]

Compromised Flaps

Current recommendations by the UHMS are to treat with HBOT at 2 ATAs to 2.5 ATAs for 90 minutes to 120 minutes. Initial treatments are given twice daily until the flap is stable; then the treatments can be reduced to daily.[24]

SUMMARY

This article is not intended to be an exhaustive defense for the use of hyperbaric oxygen as an adjunct to surgery. In truth, this has been done far better elsewhere by many of the investigators referenced in this article.[14,15,17,21,23–26,27,28] Instead, it is intended to provide a conceptual framework for the reconstructive and wound care surgeon to better understand the role of HBOT in the treatment of their patients and hopefully stimulate the timely initiation of hyperbaric therapy so as to have the most favorable impact on patient outcomes. The 2 models used (trichotomy of perfusion and ischemia-reperfusion) also are manifest in conditions, such as traumatic brain injury, myocardial infarction, and stroke,[16] which begin as pure ischemic insults and manifest the trichotomy of perfusion and its associated penumbra. Once blood flow is restored, however, these conditions evolve to behave like ischemia-reperfusion injury. The role of HBOT for these conditions has yet to be elucidated, although some of these conditions are the subject of multicenter studies (**Fig. 2**).

REFERENCES

1. Gesell LB. Hypebaric oxygen therapy indications. Durham (NC): Undersea and Hyperbaric Medical Society; 2008.
2. Weaver LK. Carbon monoxide poisoning: in hyperbaric oxygen therapy indications. Durham (NC): Undersea and Hyperbaric Medical Society; 2008.
3. Thom SR, Meyers RAM, Kindwall EP. Carbon monoxide and cyanide poisoning in hyperbaric medicine. In: Kindwall EP, Whelan HT, editors. Hyperbaric Medicine Practice. 3rd" edition. Flagstaff (AZ): Best Publishing Company; 2008.
4. Thom SR. Functional inhibition of leukocyte B2 integrins by hyperbaric oxygen in carbon monoxide-mediated brain injury in rats. Toxicol Appl Pharmacol 1993; 123:248–56.
5. Thom SR, Mendiguren I, Hardy KR, et al. Inhibition of human neutrophil beta 2 integrin-dependent adherence by hyperbaric oxygen. Am J Physiol 1997;272: C770–7.
6. Moon RE. Decompression illness: in hyperbaric oxygen therapy indications. Durham (NC): Undersea and Hyperbaric Medical Society; 2008.
7. Elliot DH, Kindwall EP. Decompression illness in hyperbaric medicine. In: Kindwall EP, Whelan HT, editors. Hyperbaric Medicine Practice. 3rd" edition. Flagstaff (AZ): Best Publishing Company; 2008.
8. Eckenhoff RG, Olstad CS, Carrod G. Human dose-response relationship for decompression and endogenous bubble formation. J Appl Physiol 1990;63(3): 914–8.
9. Philp RB, Schacham P, Gowdy CW. Involvement of platelets and microthrombi in experimental decompression sickness: similarities with disseminated intravascular coagulation. Aerosp Med 1971;42:494–502.
10. Helps SC, Gorman DF. Air embolism of the brain in rabbits pre-treated with mechlorethamine. Stroke 1991;22:351–4.
11. Madden LA, Laden G. Gas bubbles may not be the underlying cause of decompression illness - The at-depth endothelial dysfunction hypothesis. Medical Hypothesis 2009;72:389–92.
12. Martin JD, Thom SR. Vascular leukocyte sequestration in decompression sickness and prophylactic hyperbaric oxygen in rats. Aviat Space Environ Med 2002;73(6):565–9.
13. Nosum V, Hjelde A, Brubakk AO. Small amounts of venous gas embolism cause delayed impairment of endothelial function and increase polymorphonuclear neutrophil infiltration. Eur J Appl Physiol 2002;86:209–14.
14. Zamboni WA, Roth AC, Russell RC, et al. The effect of hyperbaric oxygen treatment on the microcirculation of ischemic skeletal muscle. Undersea Biomed Reseacch 1990;17(suppl):26 (abstract).

15. Strauss MB. Crush injuries and skeletal muscle-compartment syndromes: in hyperbaric oxygen therapy indications. Durham (NC): Undersea and Hyperbaric Medical Society; 2008.
16. Francis A, Baynosa R. Ischemia-reperfusion injury and hyperbaric oxygen pathways: a review of cellular mechanisms. Diving Hyperb Med 2017;47(2):110–7.
17. Nylander G, Lewis D. Reduction of post ischemic edema with hyperbaric oxygen. Plast Reconstr Surg 1985;76(4):596–603.
18. Sheffield PJ. Tissue oxygen measurements with respect to soft-tissue wound healing with normobaric and hyperbaric oxygen. HBO Rev 1985;6:18–46.
19. Marx RE. Radiation injury to tissue. In: Kindwall EP, Whelan HT, editors. Hyperbaric Medicine Practice, 3rd" edition. Flagstaff (AZ): Best Publishing Company; 2008. p851–904.
20. Demling RH. Burns and other thermal injuries. In: Way LW, Doherty GM, editors. Current surgical diagnosis and treatment. 11th edition. Mcgraw-Hill Companies; 2003. p. 267.
21. Cianci P, Slade BJ. Acute thermal burn injury: in hyperbaric oxygen therapy indications. Durham (NC): Undersea and Hyperbaric Medical Society; 2008.
22. Ward PA, Till GO. The autodestructive consequences of thermal injury. J Burn Care Rehabil 1985;6:251–5.
23. Cianci P, Slade JB, Sato RM, et al. Adjunctive hyperbaric oxygen therapy in the treatment of thermal burns. Undersea Hyperb Med 2013;40(1):89–108.
24. Zamboni WA, Baynosa RC. Compromised grafts and flaps: in hyperbaric oxygen therapy indications. Durham (NC): Undersea and Hyperbaric Medical Society; 2008.
25. Zamboni WA, Roth AC, Russel RC, et al. Morphological analysis of the microcirculation during reperfusion of ischemic skeletal muscle and the effect of hyperbaric oxygen. Plast Reconstr Surg 1993;91:1110–23.
26. Hong JP, Kwon H, Chung YK, et al. The effect of hyperbaric oxygen on ischemia-reperfusion injury: an experimental study in a rat musculocutaneous flap. Ann Plast Surg 2003;51:478–87.
27. Gonnering RS, Kindwall EP, Goldmann RW. Adjunct hyperbaric oxygen therapy in periorbital reconstruction. Arch Ophthalmol 1986;104:439–43.
28. Waterhouse MA, Zamboni WA, Brown RE, et al. The use of HBO in compromised free tissue transfer and replantation, a clinical review. Undersea Hyperb Med 1993;20(Suppl):64.

The History of Wound Healing

Tiffany Brocke, MD[a], Justin Barr, MD, PhD[b,c],*

KEYWORDS

- Wound • History • Healing • Humors • Empiricism • Surgery • Bacteria
- Antibiotics

KEY POINTS

- The history of wound care is closely linked with the history of surgery.
- From humoralism to empiricism to germ theory, the approach to wound healing over time reflects the contemporary scientific theories and pathologic understanding of the process.
- Wounds remain an area of active research and innovation by surgeon-scientists.

INTRODUCTION

Surgeons care for wounded patients. They manage both traumatic injuries and the wounds they inflict in the course of an operation. The history of wound care therefore parallels the history of surgery, and studying one reflects the trajectory of the other. Some of the earliest paleolithic findings reveal mended long-bone fractures and arrowheads lodged in ossified ribcages, demonstrating that even before the rise of civilization, healers were caring for trauma in their societies.[1] This article briefly reviews the history of wound care from ancient Egypt in approximately 1500 BCE to the modern day, organized chronologically and focused on the Western world. We explore how the treatment of wounds evolved in response to changing conceptions of physiology and pathology, and how these variations reflected the society, culture, and scientific knowledge of each particular era.

ANCIENT EGYPT

As one of the world's earliest civilizations, ancient Egyptians cared both for traumatic and surgical wounds. Their healers included magicians, priests, and lay practitioners called *swnw*, all of whom used a combination of spells, drugs, and manual interventions

a Johns Hopkins University, 2418 East Baltimore Street, Baltimore, MD 21224, USA; b Department of Surgery, Duke University, DUMC 3443, Durham, NC 27710, USA; c Department of History, Duke University, DUMC 3443, Durham, NC 27710, USA
* Corresponding author. Department of Surgery, Duke University, DUMC 3443, Durham, NC 27710.
E-mail address: justin.barr@duke.edu

Surg Clin N Am 100 (2020) 787–806
https://doi.org/10.1016/j.suc.2020.04.004
0039-6109/20/© 2020 Elsevier Inc. All rights reserved.

to treat patients.[2] The *swnw* represent the rough equivalent of physicians in ancient Egypt and practiced rational medicine. They created wounds while lancing boils, draining abscesses, and circumcising genitalia.[1,2] The Edwin Smith Papyrus, written at approximately 1500 BCE, is an Egyptian textbook on the characterization and management of traumatic wounds. The injuries discussed were grouped by the anatomic structure in question, suggesting that the unknown author prioritized anatomic location over the mechanism of injury, chronicity, color, or other feature.[3] Practitioners used this article to guide management by attempting to cure their patients through the restoration of normal anatomy, such as by suturing ear wounds and reducing fractures and dislocations. Although the Egyptians had no intellectual concept of contagion, they did maintain clean dressings with daily changes. The *swnw* further treated wounds with specialized topical ointments, such as ostrich shell to stop bone bleeding and willow to draw out the heat. The ancient Egyptians thus provide one of the earliest written records of a phylogeny of wounds: wounds were sorted by location and their concerning sequelae cataloged; specific treatments were then indicated for particular features of the damaged tissue.

GRECO-ROMAN WORLD

Inaugurating Western medicine through the works of Hippocrates and Galen, Greco-Roman medicine remains best known for its promulgation of the humoral system. Although the 4 humors mostly reflected internal diseases, Greco-Roman medicine also addressed the omnipresent wounds incurred in both the constant military conflict as well as in rural civilian life (**Fig. 1**). Several tracts within the Hippocratic Corpus address treating wounds, including the text *Fractures*, with its detailed descriptions of maneuvers and mechanisms to reduce broken bones and dislocated joints.[4] Roman encyclopedist Celsus (100 CE) provides the first detailed description of arrow wounds, including a novel instrument, the spoon of Diocles, to remove them. Celsus and Galen both outlined step-by-step methods to stop bleeding, ranging from elevating the limb to direct pressure to various styptics; vessel ligation was presented as a last resort, usually using flax or linen suture. Given their belief in humors, bleeding held particular salience and commanded a great deal of attention in medical texts. Inflammation, although recognized as a part of wound healing, attracted far less writing.[5]

Although the Greeks never appeared to develop a formal military-medical system, the Roman Army had renowned, professional service. *Medici*, albeit with uneven, nonstandardized training, staffed each legion to provide wound care in the *valetudinaria*, or field hospitals, that dotted the frontiers of the Roman empire.[6] Archeological expeditions have unearthed troves of surgical instruments at these facilities, although few written descriptions of operations remain.[7] Their care consisted of efforts to arrest bleeding and restore function, with successful interventions mostly limited to superficial and/or musculoskeletal pathology.

In addition to their medical significance, wounds in the Greco-Roman world had great cultural importance, particularly in defining the hero. This trend is first evident in the *Iliad*, a war story that features detailed, and anatomically accurate, descriptions of more than 200 specific injuries.[8] Although few verses address treatment, multiple sections portray the ideal of heroic wounding: injuries sustained in hand-to-hand combat while facing the enemy and endured with nary a whimper. This idea of heroic wounding reached its apogee with Alexander the Great, who was wounded at least 7 times during his military campaigns, including a sword slash to his thigh, an arrow through his shoulder, multiple arrow wounds to his legs, and another arrow in his

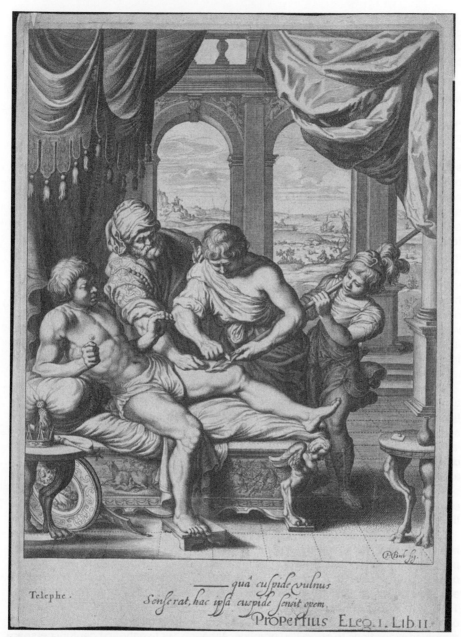

Telephe.

*quá cuspide vulnus
Senserat, hac ipsa cuspide sensit opem.*
Propertius Eleg.1.Lib.11.

Fig. 1. Early modern depiction of Greco-Roman wound care. Seventeenth century engraving by Pierre Brebiette depicting what ancient Greco-Roman wound care might have been like. Telephus (son of Hercules) is cured of a potentially fatal wound from Achilles' spear. (*Courtesy of* Wellcome collection, London, UK. Available at: https://wellcomecollection.org/works/cga3j2gq.)

chest. Contemporary biographies highlighted these wounds to demonstrate Alexander's toughness, his courage in battle, and his heroic qualities, providing a model for Greeks and Romans to emulate. This cultural association with wounds and heroism continued in the Middle Ages through the Arthurian legends and concepts of chivalry.[5]

MIDDLE AGES (CIRCA 500 CE–1453)

Although the Roman empire fell in 476 CE, Greco-Roman medicine and its humoral system remained the foundation of Western medicine for another thousand years.[9] Theory and practice differed over the centuries and from country to country, but scholars agree on some broad trends in wound care. As the medical field slowly professionalized, a distinction arose between physicians, who cared for internal diseases (the so-called natural elements), and surgeons, who held responsibility for managing wounds and diseases affecting the exterior of the body (predominately the contra-naturals) (**Fig. 2**).[10] Training for this emerging class of professional surgeons formalized over the centuries and, at the highest level, increasingly involved university education.[11] This academic background was important in an era that believed external wounds also upset the balance of the 4 humors, requiring a combined approach of local wound management along with systemic treatment.[12] It is important to note, however, that the vast majority of injured patients lacked access to formal physicians or surgeons and most likely sought attention from irregular local practitioners, from whom we have few preserved records. Paleopathological investigations do reveal a significant number of healed fractures in the skeletal remains of men and women from this era, implying reasonably effective orthopedic management from, most likely, lay healers.[13]

Formal texts described multiple ways of healing and dressing wounds. There were almost as many variations as there were authors, and they differed little from the practices of the ancient world. Wounds were washed, often with wine, and dressed. Most surgeons would apply topical medicaments like myrrh, frankincense, and honey, the latter preventing dressings from adhering to the wound. Although some texts described suturing wounds, almost no one recommended primary closure as a rule, and wounds were left to heal by what we now call secondary intention.[14,15] Regardless of their preferred treatment, surgeons in the Middle Ages spent significant time and energy thinking and writing about wound care, demonstrating its central role in both their research and daily practice.

From a modern perspective, one of the more interesting medieval wound care debates centered on the importance of laudable pus. This idea, heralding from Galen, promoted the extravasation of pus as necessary for proper wound healing, a notion quite contrary to our understanding but widely accepted at the time. Not all surgeons acceded to this doctrine, with famous medieval surgeons Henri de Mondeville and Theodoric of Lucca strongly opposed. Theodoric went so far as to assert that the provocation of pus was "the greatest possible error" in treating wounds. They, however, remained exceptions to prevailing practice. Although our twenty-first century perspective may want to criticize these forebearers for desiring what seems to be counterproductive, historian Michael McVaugh argues that in an era when almost no wound healed by primary intention, surgeons anticipated that pus would develop in every case. As such, surgeons were relieved to see it drain from the wound, so-called laudable pus, rather than risk it festering inside.[11,16]

Similar to the *Iliad* and accounts of Alexander the Great from antiquity, wounds held an important cultural role in the Middle Ages for helping define the hero. Tales of King Arthur's knights frequently recount the sword blows and arrow shots they suffered,

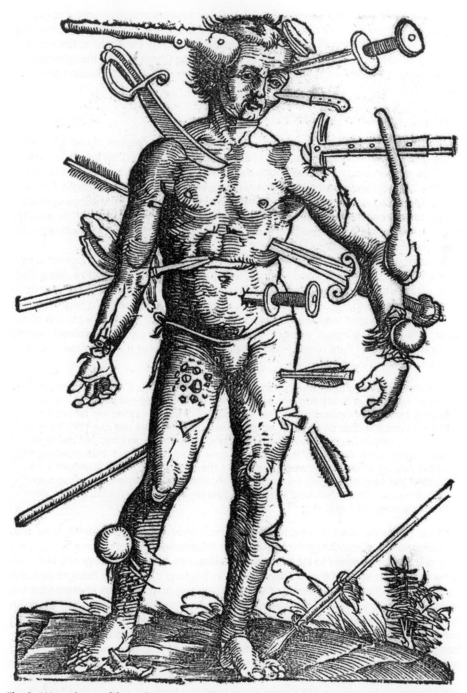

Fig. 2. Wound man, fifteenth century. Variations of "wound man" were commonly included in medieval and early modern medical texts to demonstrate the range of pathologies surgeons managed. (*Courtesy of* Wellcome collection, London, UK. Available at: https://wellcomecollection.org/works/yaw4kj5k.)

always stoically and always from the front.[17] Other paeans praised knights' ability not only to endure wounds but also to treat and heal themselves, highlighting the heroism inherent in their suffering.[18] In a medieval era dominated by the Catholic Church, this courage directly appealed to the motif of the suffering Christ.[19] With the urbanization and anonymization characteristic of the Early Modern era, this idealization of heroic wounding faded from prominence.

EARLY MODERN ERA (1453–1850)

Whereas medicine in the Middle Ages was defined by interpretation of and adherence to the ancient texts of Hippocrates et alia, empiricism characterized the early modern era. This epistemology extended from astronomy (Copernicus and heliocentrism) to physics (Newton and gravity) to anatomy (Vesalius and *De Humani Corporis Fabrica*). It also applied to wound care. The surgeon Ambroise Paré and his writings epitomize empirical advances in the treatment of traumatic injuries.[20] Most famously, he used his fortuitous experience at the siege of Turin in 1537 to transform the contemporary management of gunshot wounds.

Gunshot wounds were a new pathology in the early modern era and carried a high morbidity and mortality. Surgeons struggled to manage casualties.[21] Prevailing doctrine, established by Jean de Vigo in his classic 1514 text, held that gunpowder residue poisoned the wound, resulting in irritation, suppuration, and death. To neutralize this poison, he advocated irrigating the wound with boiling oil. As Jean was one of the most well-known surgical authors of his era, this management spread rapidly throughout Europe. Paré himself was an ardent advocate of it until he ran out of oil at Turin, recalling in his memoir:

> At last my oil lacked and I was constrained to apply in its place a digestive made of yolk of eggs, oil of roses and turpentine. That night I could not sleep at my ease, fearing by lack of cauterization that I should find the wounded on whom I had failed to put the said oil dead or empoisoned, which made me rise very early to visit them, where beyond my hope, I found those upon whom I had put the digestive medicament feeling little pain, and their wounds without inflammation or swells having rested fairly well throughout the night; the others to whom I had applied the said boiling oil, I found feverish, with great pain and swelling about their wounds. Then I resolved with myself never more to burn thus cruelly poor men wounded with gunshot.[22]

Other surgeons quickly adopted Paré's technique. More importantly, they also adopted Paré's methodology: try treatments recommended in the textbooks, but if they fail, do not be afraid to innovate and develop new therapies. Surgeons like Guillame Dupuytren in France and John Hunter in England carried this thought-process furthest, promoting a new brand of scientific surgery that came to characterize the nineteenth century. At the highest level of the profession, elective operations for aneurysms (ligation), bladder stones, and some cancers became more common, forcing practitioners to confront the consequences of iatrogenic incisions (**Fig. 3**). Outside urban areas, however, the training for the vast majority of practitioners continued via ad hoc relationships, and surgical healers focused on managing traumatic wounds.

At the same time the Reformation was reordering religious life in Europe, the medical profession began moving slowly away from the humoral system that had dominated theory and practice since Hippocrates. While iconoclasts like Paracelsus, who had served as a military surgeon and described a particularly elegant method of suturing rent intestines with silver wire, rejected humors outright, most physicians and surgeons proceeded more gradually.[23] This slow transition resulted in no small

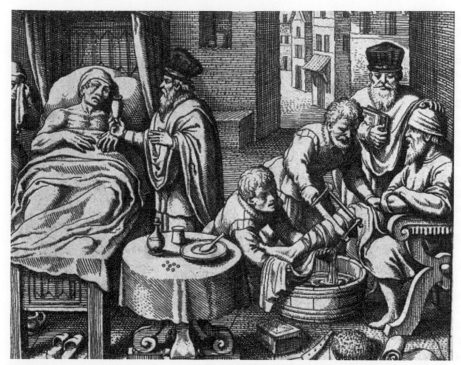

Fig. 3. Early modern medical care. This 1646 engraving shows the early modern separation of medicine (with a physician prescribing medicine on the left) and surgery (with the amputation on the right). The university-trained surgeon is standing beside the patient, supervising his assistant who is performing the operation. Note that no tourniquet controlled intraoperative blood loss, a technology not commonly used until after Petit's 1718 invention of the screw tourniquet. (*Courtesy of* Wellcome collection, London, UK. Available at: https://wellcomecollection.org/works/hm4hzfyc.)

part because none of the suggested alternatives (eg, solidism, vitalism, iatrochemistry, iatrophysics, neo-humoralism) completely explained health and disease. However, surgeons continued to believe that wounds had both local and systemic effects. Many eighteenth-century surgeons commented on the decline suffered by patients after wounding, whether by trauma or by the surgeon. John Hunter opined that the body sympathized with the wounded part[24]; his student Astley Cooper defined it as a constitutional irritation; and George James Guthrie described a constitutional alarm. The French surgeon Henri LeDran had said the body suffered a jar (*secousse*), which John Sparrow translated as *shock* in 1740.[25] What exactly caused wound shock and how to treat it became a topic of active investigation for the next 300 years.

NAPOLEONIC AND AMERICAN CIVIL WARS

Wars provided the opportunity to study wounds *en masse*, and by the nineteenth century, established military-medical systems were in place to examine casualties in a formal, systematic manner. The Napoleonic Wars (1793–1815) dominated the early decades of the nineteenth century; losses exceeded 3 million Europeans. Like all previous conflicts, deaths from disease far outnumbered combat fatalities, but traumatic wounds still numbered in the hundreds of thousands, caused predominately by small arms fire.[26] Wounds to the cranial, thoracic, and abdominal cavities were generally treated expectantly.

Surgeons in the Napoleonic Wars concentrated their attention on extremity injuries. Elective amputation provided the mainstay of therapy. The circular technique, which emerged from unknown origins in the early eighteenth century, predominated, and it presumed healing by secondary intention.[27] Without the necessity of constructing flaps or closing the wounds, surgeons recorded exceptionally fast operative times, with the famous French surgeon Dominique Jean Larrey able to remove arms and legs in well under a minute, allegedly completing 200 amputations in 24 hours after the Battle of Borodino in Russia.[28,29] Doctors controlled vessels with ligation, a therapy proposed by Celsus (100 CE), famously promulgated by Paré (1552), but not commonly used until Jean Petit's invention of the screw tourniquet (1718) that controlled hemorrhage intraoperatively.[27] Before the Napoleonic Wars, surgeons usually delayed amputation as long as possible in hopes of saving the limb. But wartime experience demonstrated the risks of systemic effects when retaining a wounded extremity, prompting the widespread adoption of early, primary amputation.

After the war, thousands of surgeons trained on the battlefields of Talavera, Borodino, and Waterloo returned to their civilian communities where they brought their military experience to bear.[30] Timing fortuitously aligned with the dawn of the Industrial Revolution, which saw millions of peasants teem into cities for perilous jobs at factories and in mines. It is impossible to determine if the number of injuries actually increased in the Industrial Revolution–farming and rural life had more than their fair share of dangers–or if the concentration of potential patients in enlarging cities attracted more medical attention, but an entire specialty of industrial medicine developed in the late nineteenth century, with factories and railroad companies hiring surgeons to manage the omnipresent wounds among their workers.[31,32] Having lost their social network of support after moving into cities, patients increasingly relied on hospitals, which expanded rapidly in number, size, and volume.[33] London's Charing Cross Hospital, for example, treated more than 66,000 traumatic injuries between 1834 and 1850; other facilities published similar statistics.[34]

The introduction of anesthesia in the 1840s facilitated treatment.[35] It made therapy less painful, leading to an increase in the number of elective operations.[34] But in the early years after its introduction, surgeons also questioned whether the elimination of pain actually hindered the healing process, prompting a complicated and uneven application of anesthesia. The rush to amputate generated by the Napoleonic Wars slowed in postwar years, as practitioners had more time to spend on each individual patient. Also, physicians like Hanoverian Georg Louis Stromeyer and the Russian military surgeon Nikolai Ivanovich Pirogov demonstrated the ability of conservative management to heal even compound fractures, helping drive a movement of limb conservation, further promoted by the introduction of plaster of Paris in 1851.[36,37] Finally, expanded access to cadavers and more regimented training curricula improved the education of clinicians managing wounds, particularly in Europe. The Europeans also had the benefit of learning lessons from the American Civil War, without having to fight in it.

Between 1861 and 1865, the Union and Confederate Armies confronted each other across the United States, with hundreds of thousands of resulting wounds. Like the Napoleonic Wars, intracavity injuries received little more than conservative management: 89% of patients with abdominal wounds in the Civil War died.[38] Medicine had little to offer these patients. But unlike the Napoleonic Wars, doctors now had anesthesia, which they used liberally. Only 254 of the documented 80,000 operations on Union soldiers proceeded without anesthesia.[39] (Most Confederate medical records burned in Richmond in 1865, limiting analysis of their side.[40]) More than 30,000 of these operations were limb amputations, which carried approximately a 25% mortality rate, half of that which the Europeans achieved in the Crimean War.[39] Surgeons had come to prefer the flap technique, implying at least the hope of healing by primary intention. Recognizing the severe social consequences amputees faced in nineteenth century America, some surgeons began trying more conservative intervention (**Fig. 4**), as recalled by J. Collins Warren, who served in the Medical Corps at the Battle of Cold Harbor: "in gunshot injuries of the joints resection of the injured ends of the bones quite often enabled the surgeon to save the limb, and this operation was regarded at the time as one of the greatest contributions to the surgery of the day."[41]

Whether amputation or a more limited bone resection, wounds festered. Although Civil War physicians did not yet recognize the germ theory, they did realize that gangrene and erysipelas were decimating their postoperative patients, and that these diseases seemed to spread from patient to patient. Doctors tried desperately to halt these mini-epidemics, trying various modes of isolation and dressings, including the including application of antiseptic solutions like bromine.[42] Nothing seemed to work consistently. These wounds also hurt. Relevant to the opioid epidemic today, doctors in the Civil War tried to control pain with subcutaneous injections of morphine, which was a recent invention. Hypodermic syringes were developed in the 1840s, and Friedrich Sertümer isolated morphine, which he named

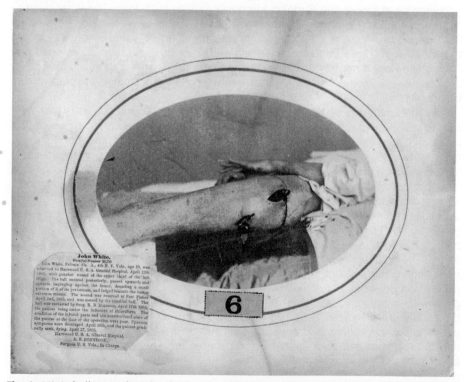

Fig. 4. Minie ball wound to the thigh. John White was 21 years old when he was wounded in the thigh during the assault on Fort Fisher; he succumbed to his wounds. (*Courtesy of* National Library of Medicine, Bethesda, MD. Available at: http://resource.nlm.nih.gov/101574218.)

after Morpheus, the Greek god of dreams, in 1804.[43,44] The mass use of morphine in the Civil War resulted in an epidemic of "soldier's disease," with more than 400,000 opioid addicts in post-bellum America, foreshadowing the social catastrophe (and the role of surgeons promulgating it) present today.[45]

LATE NINETEENTH CENTURY: CELLS, GERMS, AND ANTISEPSIS

For all the opportunities anesthesia and the Civil War unleashed, patients still died of their wounds at inexorable rates. Physicians recognized it rarely resulted from intraoperative technique but rather the postoperative suppuration. At St. Bartholomew's Hospital in England, for example, more than 40% of patients requiring an amputation died. In Paris, 52% of patients perished following major limb amputation.[46] Not fully understanding the etiology of this suppuration, doctors tried a variety of interventions ranging from isolation to smaller incisions to washing wounds; none worked consistently.[47] The solution ultimately relied on the understanding and accepting the germ theory of disease.

Germs, or more accurately, microscopic animalcules, had been visible at least since Antoni van Leeuwenhoek perfected the single-lens microscope in the late 1600s. But they appeared to be everywhere with little connection to either health or disease, and the medical profession as a whole largely ignored microscopy for 2 centuries. Advances in technology, particularly Joseph Lister's (the father) invention of the achromatic lens, permitted more exacting studies and eventually led to Theodor Schwann's cell theory and Rudolph Virchow's cellular pathology. The latter demonstrated that inflammation resulted from the accumulation of white blood cells rather than alleged neo-humors.[48] Although important theoretically, these advances did little to benefit wound care clinically. Scientists and physicians, such as Louis Pasteur in France and Robert Koch in Germany, began exploring the role of germs in the causation of disease in the late nineteenth century, offering vaccines as prophylactic treatments.[49]

Joseph Lister, son of the aforementioned microscopist and an unusually well-trained surgeon practicing in Edinburgh, faced the practical implications of this research.[50] Like his contemporaries, he searched for ways to limit postoperative mortality. In the 1860s, Lister absorbed the discoveries of Louis Pasteur, applied them to surgery, and created his antiseptic system. Convinced that microorganisms caused wound infection and that such creatures lived everywhere, in the air, on hands, on instruments, and so forth, Lister devised a system to eradicate them through dressings soaked in carbolic acid. He first applied this treatment in 1865 on James Greenlees, a young boy with a compound femur fracture. When carbolic acid dressings seemingly prevented infection in Greenlees, Lister experimented with it in other patients; 9 of his first 12 attempts healed without evidence of suppuration. He published his first article documenting this antiseptic method of treatment in the *Lancet* in March 1867. He later expanded from treating traumatic wounds to applying his technique to elective surgery, with excellent results (**Fig. 5**). Lister published dozens of modifications over the course of his lifetime. Despite the apparent success, the methodology took decades to achieve widespread acceptance.[51] But by the 1880s, antiseptic technique, and the German variant of asepsis, had become the standard method of treating both traumatic and iatrogenic wounds.

WORLD WAR I

World War I was the first major military engagement following the widespread adoption of the germ theory of disease. Research had furthered contemporaries'

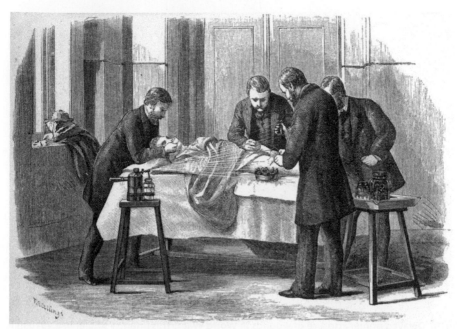

Fig. 5. Early antiseptic surgery. A spray of carbolic acid douses the open wound and hands of the surgeons while towels soaked in carbolic acid surround the edges of the incision; instruments sit in a bowl of carbolic acid in the foreground. Note the use of chloroform anesthesia. (*Courtesy of* Wellcome collection, London, UK. Available at: https://wellcomecollection.org/works/wdp236ft.)

understanding of wound healing. Paul Friedrich's studies of the late nineteenth century showed that it required roughly 6 hours for germs in a wound to enter the bloodstream and cause systemic detriment, providing the theoretic rationale behind early surgery.[52] Elective operations had expanded to included neuro, thoracic, and intraabdominal surgery.[53] Surgeons entered World War I excited about their potential to care for combat casualties; the mass destruction of war and millions of wounded soldiers diminished their sanguine enthusiasm but ultimately led to new modalities of managing wounds.[54]

World War I, chiefly fought in the manure-fertilized fields of northern Europe, created filthy wounds that teemed with microorganisms. The conservative management of gunshot wounds that proved so effective in the Boer and Russo-Japanese War, where surgeons dressed but did not operate on penetrating trauma, failed miserably in Europe, as thousands of casualties died of gangrene and other presumably preventable infections.[55,56] Two solutions materialized. First, pioneering surgeons like H.M.W. Gray in the British Army and Antoine DePage in the Belgian military recognized the importance of keeping fresh wounds open with delayed primary closure, removing all foreign bodies, and extirpating any necrotic or devascularized tissue, a process dubbed debridement (**Fig. 6**).[57,58] By 1917, debridement became standard of care and extended from soft tissue injuries to include the management of cranial trauma and exploratory laparotomies for abdominal wounds.[59–61]

Second, surgeons realized that not even the most thorough debridement could eradicate all germs. With asepsis impossible, they returned to Listerian antisepsis

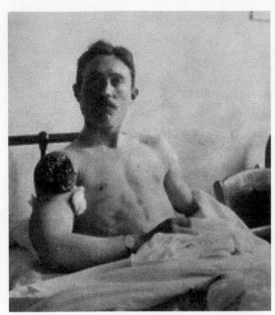

Fig. 6. Delayed primary closure of wounds in World War I. This infantry soldier in a 1916 military hospital in France has a shoulder wound that was treated with delayed primary closure. (*Courtesy of* Wellcome collection, London, UK. Available at: https://wellcomecollection.org/works/hn9jdmkk.)

by dousing wounds with various chemicals. Although multiple alternatives existed, the Carrel-Dakin system was the most common.[62,63] Nobel Prize–winning surgeon Alexis Carrel worked with Rockefeller chemist Henry Dakin, who invented an antiseptic treatment consisting of a solution of sodium hypochlorite buffered to physiologic pH: Dakin's solution. Carrel designed a series of fenestrated catheters to distribute the solution evenly through the wound bed. Anecdotally at least, the Carrel-Dakin system significantly reduced the rates of infection, and it remained the standard of care for treating septic wounds until the arrival of penicillin in the 1940s. Dakin's solution continues to be used for contaminated wounds in both military and civilian patients.[64]

In addition to the local effects of wounds and subsequent infectious complications, military doctors tried to address the physiologic disarray that accompanied the trauma: the "shock" that LeDran had identified centuries earlier. Research since Le Dran had tried to determine its etiology and came up with a number of possibilities ranging from George Crile's theory of vasomotor malfunction causing venous dilation to Walter B. Cannon's idea that acidosis resulted in blood pooling in the abdomen.[25] Surgeons on the frontline noted that "although physiologists have for years past been trying to define shock for us, we clinicians are fairly well agreed upon the matter," diagnosing patients based on tachycardia, hypotension, tachypnea, and altered mental status.[65] Treatments varied but centered on keeping the patient warm and dry. Many doctors attempted fluid resuscitation through saline enemata, subcutaneous injections, and intravenous boli of both crystalloid and colloid solutions, although in volumes (typically less than 1 L) that in retrospect explained their relative inefficacy.

ANTIBIOTICS AND WORLD WAR II

Pasteur's germ theory and Lister's antisepsis and asepsis marked a new era in rational wound care that, by the mid-twentieth century led directly to the next great advance: antibiosis. While Alexander Fleming discovered the mold penicillin in 1928, Prontosil (1934), a sulfa drug, was the first clinically relevant antibiotic used to treat wounds.[66,67] It quickly proved effective against the streptococci and staphylococci that physician-scientists had identified as the primary cause of cellulitis and deep-space abscesses, respectively.[68]

At the advent of World War II, the military was motivated to control wound and burn infections and quickly began to experiment with antibiotics. Results from the Spanish Civil War suggested that oral sulfonamides prevented wound infection. By 1942, it was official American military doctrine to use both oral sulfonamides and sulfa crystals directly in wounds (**Fig. 7**). This trend was fairly short-lived. A 1943 clinical study showed that neither oral nor topical sulfonamides affected rates of wound infection, and that low infection rates were attributable to surgical technique. By 1945, the Office of the Surgeon General no longer recommended sulfa powders for wounds.[67]

Penicillin promised improved results. A multi–billion-dollar joint government-industry research effort spent years working to produce the mold in sufficient quantities for its widespread use; by D-Day, there was enough to treat wounded soldiers, sailors, and Marines, although it remained exquisitely rare for civilians in the United States for another year (**Fig. 8**). In 1944, Allen O. Whipple wrote about systemic penicillin as a potent means to prevent the onset and spread of infection. As evidence, he quoted a clinical trial, the modern hybrid of Paré's observation and Galen's logic, in which penicillin combined with surgery was more likely to eliminate infections, reduce pain, and lead to more complete restoration of function. He warned that, "until the bacterial infection in the zone surrounding the infection is

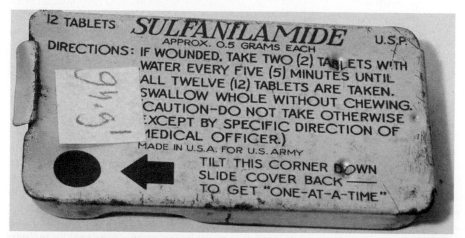

Fig. 7. Sulfa tin distributed to US Army medics in World War II. Initially, all soldiers in World War II were issued sulfa powder packs to sprinkle over wounds, although lack of efficacy led to the cessation of this practice. Medics carried sulfa tablets, also of questionable utility, and doctors used intravenous formulations, which were useful in treating a range of infections. (*Courtesy of* National Liberation Museum 1944-1945, Groesbeek, The Netherlands. Available at: https://commons.wikimedia.org/wiki/File:Can_of_12_Sulfanilamide_tablets.JPG.)

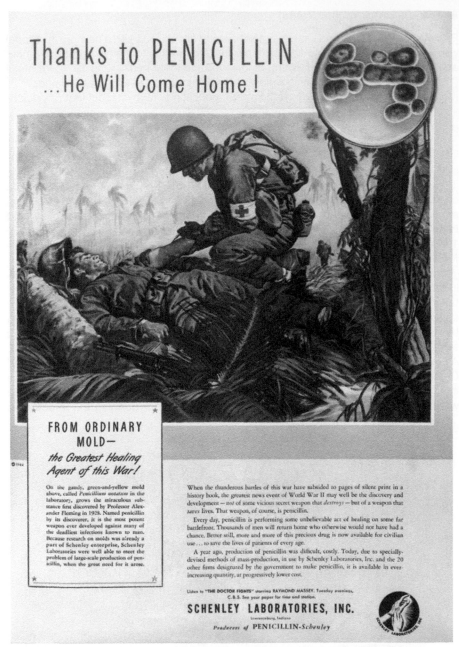

Fig. 8. Penicillin propaganda poster from World War II. Poster championing the creation and utility of penicillin. Note the Petri dish in the right upper corner, advertising that only makes sense in an era in which germ theory was widely accepted not only among doctors but also among the lay community. (*Courtesy of* Wellcome collection, London, UK. Available at: https://wellcomecollection.org/works/apnj2urs.)

controlled, [other measures to promote healing] will be ineffective," critically cautioning that antibiotics alone would not solve the issue of infection but that it required both drug therapy and surgery to heal patients, a synergy that remains essential today.[69]

Antibiotics altered the surgical and wound care landscape in many ways. For example, the specter of pulmonary tuberculosis became treatable without resort to thoracoplasty or collapse therapy, effectively eliminating incisional wounds for that disease.[70] However, the early indiscriminate use of antibiotics and the subsequent microbial resistance patterns that developed changed which infections threatened patients.[71] Although the once-dangerous streptococcal erysipelas and cellulitis remained susceptible to sulfonamides, *Staphylococcus* has become rapidly drug-resistant, spawning new challenges for physicians and surgeons that may soon resemble those of the early nineteenth century.[68,72]

POSTWAR WOUND THERAPY

Whipple's writing demonstrates that by 1944, the medical understanding of wounds had changed to a form we recognize today. A wound was still the "loss of continuity of tissues," but the tissues in question were now individual cells, each known to have a role in healing. Appropriate approximation and immobilization of wounds remained important, but was understood to follow rationally from its microarchitecture. The supply of both oxygen and nutrition to tissues was augmentable through blood transfusion and total parenteral nutrition. New surgical techniques allowed for the restoration of blood to tissue through vascular anastomoses and grafts.[73] Facile tissue coverage benefited from increased use of skin grafts, which progressed dramatically after their advent in 1869.[74]

This understanding of wound biology explains the success of an ancient technology that underwent a renaissance in the late twentieth century: negative-pressure wound therapy. The ancient Egyptians and Romans provided oral suction to wounds to withdraw poisons and evil humors within. As the understanding of microbes advanced in the nineteenth century and humoral theory fell out of favor, these practices disappeared from doctors' armamentarium. Based on an entirely different understanding of pathophysiology, Louis C. Argenta and Michael Morykwas reintroduced negative-pressure wound therapy in 1997 (**Fig. 9**). Their wound vacuum was found to enhance formation of granulation tissue by removing third-spaced fluid, which decreased capillary afterload and promoted circulatory inflow to the wound.[75] It has become an omnipresent tool for managing complex wounds in the twenty-first century, although it continues to rely on fundamental principles found in the teachings of Hippocrates and Galen more than 2000 years ago.

Modern wound therapy prominently features nurses. Although nurses have been involved in wound care since the birth of the profession under Florence Nightingale, dedicated wound care nursing was born as enterostomal therapy at the Cleveland Clinic in 1958.[76] The program expanded around the body as they assumed responsibility for a broader array of pathologies as well as extending around the country as wound-care nurses became increasingly prevalent in hospitals, nursing homes, and home-health agencies. Few studies directly compare healing rates of wounds managed by physicians versus specially trained nurses versus regular nurses, but what literature does exist suggests some clinical benefit to involving these providers.[77–79] The current incarnation of wound care nursing reflects several modern trends in health care, including increased specialization as well as delegation of responsibility from physicians to other members of the health care team.

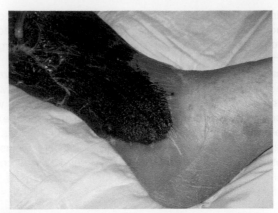

Fig. 9. Negative-pressure wound therapy. The wound vac, in use here on a diabetic foot infection, enhances the surgeon's armamentarium in the setting of modern barriers to the healing of chronic wounds. The black polyurethane sponge covers the wound bed, and plastic adhesive provides an airtight seal for the vacuum appliance seen at the upper left. (Image from Wikimedia Commons. Available at: https://commons.wikimedia.org/wiki/File:V.A.C.-Verband.jpg.)

SUMMARY

The history of wounds is the history of surgery. Wound care has evolved over time to reflect both the needs of patients and the surgeon's understanding of the pathology involved. The modern state of wound care is not the endpoint of the field. As larger societal technologies change, these patterns are reflected in changing wounds. Laparoscopic surgery has produced much smaller iatrogenic wounds, but more of them. More powerful weapons, combined with improved survivability from body armor, create devastating combat wounds.[80] Other practice patterns have changed wound care further. Surgical site infections are tracked as they have never been before in national databases like the National Surgical Quality Improvement Program and the National Cancer Database. Tied to quality benchmarks, these metrics created new incentives for research and interventions to minimize wound infection. In an era of American mass shootings, bystander interventions like Stop the Bleed are an attempt to increase layperson involvement in wound hemostasis.[81] New technologies, such as synthetic skin substitutes and hyperbaric oxygen, are under exploration for complex, nonhealing wounds (see Holly Ortman and James Abdo's article, "Biologic and Synthetic CTPs and "Smart" Wound Dressings/Coverings"; and Michael James and colleagues' article, "Defining the Role of Hyperbaric Oxygen Therapy as an Adjunct to Reconstructive Surgery," elsewhere in this issue).

Other social trends will continue to challenge surgeons attempting to manage wounds, including a patient population with a greater number and higher complexity of comorbidities (see Robel T. Beyene and colleagues' article, "The Effect of Comorbidities on Wound Healing," elsewhere in this issue). Cigarette smoking remains prevalent worldwide and is known to affect the tissue microenvironment, leading to impaired wound healing. The circulatory dysfunction and chronic inflammation of diabetes mellitus generate new and challenging wounds in patients, hindering body-wide healing (see Stephanie R. Goldberg and Robert F. Diegelmann's article, "What Makes Wounds Chronic"; and Robel T. Beyene and colleagues' article, "The Effect of Comorbidities on Wound Healing"; and Christopher Bibbo and colleagues' article, "Foot and Ankle Surgery for Chronic Non-healing Wounds," elsewhere in this issue).[82] As an increasing number of implantable devices are approved for medical use, the problem of biofilms in healing has mounted as well (see Steven R. Evelhoch's article, "Biofilm and Chronic Non-Healing Wound Infections," elsewhere in this issue). Perhaps most recently, surgeons have recognized a limited understanding of how immunomodulators affect wound healing. Newer biologic medications are raising complicated questions around operative decision making, most notably with regard to the risk of colorectal anastomotic leak.[83] Despite these challenges and ever-advancing technology, the fundamental role of the surgeon in managing his or her patients' wounds remains an unchanged, challenging, and a defining feature of the profession.

DISCLOSURE

None.

REFERENCES

1. Majno G. The healing hand: man and his wound in the ancient world. Cambridge (England): Harvard University Press; 1975.
2. Estes JW. The medical skills of Ancient Egypt. Revised edition. Canton (MA): Science Hill Publications; 1993.
3. Sanchez GM, Meltzer ES. Edwin Smith papyrus: updated translation of the trauma treatise and modern medical commentaries. Atlanta (GA): Lockwood Press; 2012.
4. Milne JS. The apparatus used by the Greeks and Romans in the setting of fractures and the reduction of dislocations. Interstate Medical Journal Company 1909;16:48–60.
5. Salazar CF. The treatment of war wounds in Graeco-Roman Antiquity. Boston: Brill; 2000.
6. Davies RW. The Roman Military Medical Service. In: Breeze DJ, Maxfield VA, editors. Service in the Roman Army. Edinburgh: Edinburgh University Press; 1989. p. 209–30.
7. Baker PA. Medical care of the Roman Army on the Rhine, Danube and British frontiers in the first, second and early third centuries AD. BAR International Series; 2004.
8. Adamson P. A comparison of ancient and modern weapons in the effectiveness of producing battle casualties. J R Army Med Corps. 1977;123(2):93–103.
9. Siraisi NG. Medieval and early renaissance medicine. Chicago: University of Chicago Press; 1990.
10. Demaitre LE. Medieval medicine: the art of healing, from head to toe. Denver (CO): Praeger; 2013.
11. McVaugh M. The rational surgery of the middle ages. Sismel: Firenzae Press; 2006.
12. Naylor I. Medicine for surgical practice in fourteenth-century England: the judgment against John le Spicer. In: Kirkham A, Warr C, editors. Wounds in the middle ages. Burlington (VT): Ashgate; 2014. p. 175–95.
13. Aufderheide AC. The Cambridge encyclopedia of human paleopathology. Boston: Credo Reference; 2014.
14. Clasper J. The management of military wounds in the middle ages. In: Kirkham A, Warr C, editors. Wounds in the middle ages. Burlington (VT): Ashgate; 2004. p. 17–39.

15. van't Land K. The solution of continuous things: wounds in late medeival mediine and surgery. In: Kirkham A, Warr C, editors. Wounds in the middle ages. Burlington (VT): Ashgate; 2004. p. 89–108.
16. Cartwright FF. The development of modern surgery. New York: T.Y. Crowell; 1968.
17. Gould GM, Pyle WL. King Arthur's medicine. Bulletin of the Johns Hopkins Hospital; 1897. VIII(8):239–46.
18. Priest H. Christ's wounds and the birth of romance. In: Kirkham A, Warr C, editors. Wounds in the middle ages. Burlington (VT): Ashgate; 2014. p. 131–50.
19. Amundsen DW. Medicine, society, and faith in the ancient and medieval worlds. Baltimore: Johns Hopkins University Press; 1996.
20. Hamby WB. Ambroise Paré: surgeon of the renaissance. St. Louis (MO): Warren H. Green, Inc; 1967.
21. Billroth T. Historical studies on the nature and treatment of gunshot wounds from the fifteenth century to the present time. Yale J Biol Med 1931;4:1932;4.
22. Paré A. The apologie and treatise of ambroise pare. Birmingham (Al): Classics of Medicine Library; 1984.
23. Webster C. Paracelsus: medicine, magic, and mission at the end of time. New Haven (CT): Yale University Press; 2008.
24. Hunter J. A treatise on the blood, inflammation, and gun-shot wounds. London: 1794.
25. English PC. Shock, physiological surgery, and George Washington crile: medical innovation in the progressive era. Westport (CT): Greenwood Press; 1980.
26. Crumplin M. Men of steel: surgery in the Napoleonic Wars. Shrewsbury (England): Quiller Press; 2007.
27. Kirkup J. A history of limb amputation. London: Springer; 2007.
28. Skandalakis PN, Lainas P, Zoras O, et al. "To Afford the Wounded Speedy Assistance": Dominique Jean Larrey and Napoleon. World J Surg 2006;30(8):1392–9.
29. Dible JH. Napoleon's surgeon. London: Heinemann; 1970.
30. Ackroyd M, Brockliss LWB, Moss M, et al. Advancing with the Army: medicine, the professions, and social mobility in the British isles, 1790-1850. New York: Oxford University Press; 2006.
31. Rutkow IM. Railway surgery: traumatology and managed health care in 19th-century United States. Arch Surg 1993;128(4):458–63.
32. Buess H. The beginnings of industrial medicine in England. Br J Ind Med 1962; 19(4):297–302.
33. Risse GB. Mending bodies, saving souls: a history of hospitals. New York: Oxford University Press; 1999.
34. Stanley P. For fear of pain: British Surgery, 1790-1850. Amsterdam: Rodopi; 2003.
35. Pernick MS. A calculus of suffering: pain, professionalism, and anesthesia in nineteenth-century America. New York: Columbia University Press; 1985.
36. Stromeyer GFL. Gunshot fractures. Philadelphia: Lippincott; 1862.
37. Smith PF. Louis Stromeyer (1804–76): German orthopaedic and military surgeon and his links with Britain. J Med Biogr 2006;14(2):65–74.
38. Gillet MC. The Army medical department 1818-1865. Washington, DC: Center of Military History; 2000.
39. Bollet AJ. Civil War medicine: challenges and triumphs. Tuscon (AZ): Galen Press, Ltd; 2002.
40. Cunningham HH. Doctors in gray: the Confederate medical service. Baton Rouge (LA): Louisiana State University Press; 1958.
41. Warren JC. To work in the vineyard of surgery. Cambridge (MA): Harvard University Press; 1958.

42. Devine S. Learning from the wounded: the Civil War and the rise of American medical science. Chapel Hill (NC): University of North Carolina Press; 2014.
43. Howard-Jones N. The origins of hypodermic medication. Sci Am 1971;224(1): 96–103.
44. Schmitz R. Friedrich Wilhelm Sertürner and the discovery of morphine. Pharm Hist 1985;27(2):61–74.
45. Courtwright DT. Dark paradise: opiate addiction in America before 1940. Cambridge (MA): Harvard Univerity Press; 1982.
46. Wangensteen OH, Wangensteen SD, Klinger C. Surgical cleanliness, hospital salubrity, and surgical statistics, historically considered. Surgery 1972;71(4): 477–93.
47. Kernahan PJ. Causation and cleanliness: George Callender, wounds, and the debates over listerism. J Hist Med Allied Sci 2009;64(1):1–37.
48. Ackerknecht EH. Rudolf Virchow: doctor, statesman, anthropologist. Madison (WI): University of Wisconsin Press; 1953.
49. Carter KC. The rise of causal concepts of disease: case histories. Burlington (VT): Ashgate; 2003.
50. Godlee RJ. Lord Lister. London: Macmillan; 1917.
51. Gariepy TP. The introduction and acceptance of listerian antisepsis in the United States. J Hist Med Allied Sci 1994;49(2):167–206.
52. Friedrich PL. Die aseptische versorgung frischer wundern. Archiv fur Klinische Chirurgie 1898;57:288–310.
53. Wangensteen OD, Wangensteen SA. The rise of surgery: from empiric craft to scientific discipline. Minneapolis (MN): University of Minnesota Press; 1978.
54. Barr J, Cancio LC, Smith DJ, et al. From trench to bedside: military surgery during World War I upon its centennial. Mil Med 2019;184(11–12):214–20.
55. Makins GH. Surgical experiences in South Africa, 1899-1900; being mainly a clinical study of the nature and effects of injuries produced by bullets of small calibre. 2nd edition. London: Frowde; 1913.
56. Barr J. Military medicine of the Russo-Japanese war and its influence on the modernization of the US Army Medical Department. US Army Med Dep J 2016;(3–16):118–28.
57. Harrison M. The medical war: British military medicine in World War I. Oxford: Oxford University Press; 2010.
58. Helling TS, Daon E. Flanders fields: the Great War, Antoine Depage, and the resurgence of debridement. Ann Surg 1998;228(2):173–81.
59. Cushing H. From a surgeon's journal: 1915-1918. Boston: Little, Brown, and Company; 1936.
60. Currie D. Wounds of the Skull and Brain. In: Scotland TR, Hays S, editors. War surgery 1914-1918. Solihull (England: Helion and Co; 2012. p. 234–56.
61. Bamberger PK. The adoption of laparotomy for the treatment of penetrating abdominal wounds in war. Mil Med 1996;161(4):189–96.
62. Haller JS Jr. Treatment of infected wounds during the Great War, 1914 to 1918. South Med J 1992;85(3):303–15.
63. Carrel A, Dehelly G. Le Traitment des Plaies Infectées. Paris: Masson et Cie; 1917.
64. Cannon JW, Hofmann LJ, Glasgow SC, et al. Dismounted complex blast injuries: a comprehensive review of the modern combat experience. J Am Coll Surg 2016; 223(4):652–64.e8.
65. Archibald EW, McLean W. Observations upon shock, with particular reference to the condition as seen in war surgery. Ann Surg 1917;66(3):280–6.

66. Bud R. Penicillin: triumph and tragedy. New York: Oxford University Press; 2007.

67. Lesch JE. The first miracle drugs: how the sulfa drugs transformed medicine. New York: Oxford University Press; 2007.

68. Wangensteen OH, Wangensteen SD, Klinger CF. Wound management of Ambroise Paré and Dominique Larrey, great French military surgeons of the 16th and 19th centuries. Bull Hist Med 1972;46(3):207.

69. Whipple AO. Recent advances in the treatment of wounds. Proc Am Philos Soc 1944;88(3):177–81.

70. Herbsman H. Early history of pulmonary surgery. J Hist Med Allied Sci 1958; 13(3):329–48.

71. Podolsky SH. The antibiotic era: reform, resistance, and the pursuit of a rational therapeutics. Baltimore: Johns Hopkins University Press; 2015.

72. McKenna M. Superbug: the fatal menace of MRSA. New York: Free Press; 2010.

73. Barr J. Of life and limb: surgical repair of the arteries in war and peace, 1880-1960. Rochester (NY): University of Rochester Press; 2019.

74. Oppenheimer J. Taking things apart and putting them together again. Bull Hist Med 1978;52(2):149–61.

75. Argenta L, Morykwas M. Vacuum-assisted closure: a new method for wound control and treatment: clinical experience. Ann Plast Surg 1997;38(6):563–76.

76. Corbett LQ. Wound care nursing: professional issues and opportunities. Adv Wound Care 2012;1(5):189–93.

77. Hart S, Bergquist S, Gajewski B, et al. Reliability testing of the national database of nursing quality indicators pressure ulcer indicator. J Nurs Care Qual 2006; 21(3):256–65.

78. Zulkowski K, Ayello EA, Wexler S. Certification and education: do they affect pressure ulcer knowledge in nursing? Adv Skin Wound Care 2007;20(1):34–8.

79. Westra BL, Bliss DZ, Savik K, et al. Effectiveness of wound, ostomy, and continence nurses on agency-level wound and incontinence outcomes in home care. Home Healthc Now 2014;32(2):119–27.

80. Kellermann A, Elster E, Babington C, et al. Out of the crucible: how the US military transformed combat casualty care in Iraq and Afghanistan. Ft. Sam Houston: Office of the Surgeon General; 2018.

81. Butler FK. Stop the bleed. Strategies to enhance survival in active shooter and intentional mass casualty events. The Hartford Consensus. A major step forward in translating battlefield trauma care advances to the civilian sector. J Spec Oper Med 2015;15(4):133–5.

82. Baltzis D, Eleftheriadou I, Veves A. Pathogenesis and treatment of impaired wound healing in diabetes mellitus: new insights. Adv Ther 2014;31(8):817–36.

83. Nikolian VC, Kamdar NS, Regenbogen SE, et al. Anastomotic leak after colorectal resection: a population-based study of risk factors and hospital variation. Surgery 2017;161(6):1619–27.

Vascular Assessment of the Lower Extremity with a Chronic Wound

Jonathan F. Arnold, MD

KEYWORDS

- Ankle-brachial index • Skin perfusion pressure
- Transcutaneous oxygen pressure measurement • Near-infrared imaging

KEY POINTS

- A thorough history and physical examination of patients with chronic lower extremity wounds should be performed, including assessment of peripheral arterial disease risk in the patient's medical and surgical history, inquiry on the presence of intermittent claudication symptoms, visual assessment, and pulse palpation and auscultation. Auscultation of a femoral bruit, absence of pedal pulses, and monophasic signal on handheld Doppler examination are all concerning findings that should prompt further evaluation for PAD.

- Ankle and toe pressures and ankle and toe-brachial indices can be falsely elevated due to arterial calcification and provide vascular assessment at the level of the tourniquet only. Dividing the lower of the posterior tibial or dorsalispedis systolic pressures by the higher brachial artery to calculate the ankle-brachial index may help better identify patients with peripheral arterial disease. Variations in cut-off values for the toe-brachial index, less than 0.54 to 0.75, make it difficult to determine a proper diagnosis of peripheral vascular disease. Additional vascular studies are recommended if results are inconclusive.

- Transcutaneous oxygen pressure measurement (TCOM) and skin perfusion pressure (SPP) measurements have been reported to be better able to predict wound healing and the necessity for amputation than ankle and toe pressure measurements. Variation in cut-off values signifying adequate perfusion, 25 mmHg to 50 mmHg for TCOM and 30 mmHg to 40 mmHg and up to 70 mmHg in patients with end-stage renal disease on hemodialysis for SPP, along with need to extrapolate perfusion within the wound bed may limit their utility in accurate vascular assessment for healing.

- Hyperspectral and near-infrared image provide a means of vascular assessment not restricted by limitations of traditional vascular studies and provide the ability to assess perfusion directly within the wound bed. These modalities assess tissue oxygenation levels or local perfusion by means of a fluorescent dye. Decreased tissue oxygenation or decreased fluorescent dye in the wound bed and mottled signal appearance has been associated with peripheral arterial disease and delayed wound healing. These modalities may also assist in determining the presence of inflammation and infection in and about the wound.

Continued

Mercy Healing Center, 701 10th Street Southeast, Cedar Rapids, IA 52403, USA
E-mail address: jarnold@mercycare.org

Surg Clin N Am 100 (2020) 807–822
https://doi.org/10.1016/j.suc.2020.05.008
0039-6109/20/© 2020 Elsevier Inc. All rights reserved.
surgical.theclinics.com

Continued

- The need for quantitative and accurate information of adequate blood supply is critical for timely intervention, if necessary, in patients with a chronic wound of the lower extremity. Proper vascular assessment should include a thorough history and physical examination and combination of routine and novel vascular studies.

INTRODUCTION

Peripheral arterial disease (PAD) exists on a spectrum ranging from asymptomatic to critical limb ischemia (CLI), affecting approximately 8.5 million people older than 40 years in the United States and 202 million people worldwide.[1–4] Its presence is associated with significant morbidity and mortality related to cerebral vascular accidents and cardiovascular events.[5] Patients with diabetes with or without amputation have a 5-year mortality rate of 46% to 48%, respectively, higher than mortality rates of prostate and breast cancer combined.[6] The true incidence of PAD may be underestimated due to the number of asymptomatic patients who go undiagnosed.[5] The initial diagnostic test for PAD screening is the ankle-brachial index (ABI).[2,7] However, controversy exists in the risk versus benefit of obtaining this test in asymptomatic patients.[5,8] Yet, more than 50% of patients with PAD are asymptomatic; further complicating this are those patients in whom routine noninvasive vascular studies have limitations.[3–5,9–12] Lower extremity PAD is often not recognized until a complication presents, such as severe pain, tissue loss with delayed healing, or gangrene.[13] For these reasons, the American Heart Association/American College of Cardiology (AHA/ACC) recommend patients with known PAD and those at increased risk for PAD with history and physical examination findings that suggest PAD should undergo diagnostic testing. Patients at increased risk for PAD per the AHA/ACC are listed in **Box 1.**[4] The guidelines for management of the diabetic foot from the Society for Vascular Surgery, the American Podiatric Medical Association, and the Society for Vascular Medicine recommend an ABI be obtained in all patients with diabetes older than 50 years.[14]

Delay in revascularization in patients with lower extremity tissue loss and PAD can further propagate complications of delayed healing, infection, amputation, and death.[5] Knowledge of signs and symptoms of PAD to look for in a patient's history and

---

Box 1
Patients at increased risk for peripheral arterial disease per the American College of Cardiology/American Heart Association practice guidelines

Age ≥65 years

Age 50 to 64 years, with risk factors for atherosclerosis (eg, diabetes mellitus, history of smoking, hyperlipidemia, hypertension) or family history of peripheral arterial disease

Age less than 50 years, with diabetes mellitus and 1 additional risk factor for atherosclerosis

Individuals with known atherosclerotic disease in another vascular bed (eg, coronary, carotid, subclavian, renal, mesenteric artery stenosis, or abdominal aortic aneurysm)

From Writing Committee Members, Gerhard-Herman MD, Gornik HL, et al. 2016 AHA/ACC Guideline on the Management of Patients with Lower Extremity Peripheral Artery Disease: Executive Summary. Vasc Med. 2017;22(3):NP1–NP43; with permission.

physical examination, limitations of current noninvasive vascular studies, and novel technologies for vascular assessment can better assist the treating provider in identifying PAD in patients with a lower extremity wound and developing the optimal treatment plan for resolution. The objective of this article is to present current and novel vascular assessment technologies to assist the provider in selection of which studies would be optimal in determining vascular status and the potential need for intervention when treating a patient with a wound of the lower extremity.

LOWER EXTREMITY VASCULAR ASSESSMENT
History

Lower extremity vascular assessment begins by obtaining a thorough history and physical examination. Questions to the patient regarding the presence of risk factors for PAD, in addition to being of older age, can heighten suspicion of its potential diagnosis. African American patients are at greater risk for PAD.[13] Patients should also be asked about personal history of coronary artery disease, cerebrovascular disease, including transient ischemic attacks and strokes, hypertension, hypercholesterolemia, obesity, chronic kidney disease, and diabetes, and a family history of PAD, cardiovascular disease, and renal insufficiency.[1,5,9,13,15,16] Presence of comorbidities can also be assessed through medication list reconciliation.[1] Surgical history of previous vascular-related procedures and surgeries such as carotid, coronary, and peripheral vascular procedures should also be obtained. Social history should also be obtained in regard to normal activity levels and previous and current tobacco use, both of which are known risk factors for PAD.[1,5,9,15,16] Cigarette smoking increased the risk of PAD from 2- to 6-fold.[17] There is an increased risk for PAD in younger patients in whom the presence of the abovementioned comorbidities and social history risk factors are present.[5]

As intermittent claudication is the most common symptom associated with PAD, its presence should be questioned. Intermittent claudication is defined as reproducible discomfort in a specific muscle group of the lower extremity that occurs after a predictable level of activity, is relieved by rest, and recurs in this same fashion.[1,17,18] Questioning should discern what muscle group in the lower extremity is affected, to determine possible level of arterial lesion and quantification of the duration of activity that produces the symptom; this provides a baseline for future reference and can speak to the potential severity of the arterial lesion. Knowing if this interferes and has limited the patient's mobility also helps determine potential PAD severity.[1,18,19] Other questions geared more to rest pain and severe PAD involve asking the patient if they experience in the foot, often localized to the ball of the foot, which wakes them up at night and is relieved by dangling the foot over the side of the bed. Some patients sleep sitting up to avoid this pain.[1]

The difficulty in diagnosis of PAD based on the presence of intermittent claudication is that up to 78% of patients with PAD are asymptomatic even though they have the same risk factor profile as symptomatic patients.[3–5,9–13] The absence of symptoms is of particular concern in patients with diabetes who can remain asymptomatic until advanced stages of PAD when ischemic ulceration and/or gangrene become apparent because of peripheral neuropathy.[11,13,19–21] Development of adequate collateral circulation can also prevent symptoms of intermittent claudication from occurring.[9] Patients with diabetes should be questioned about medications taken for glycemic control, what their glycemic control is like and how often it is checked, and the duration of diagnosis.[1] Patients with diabetes have a 4- to 10-fold increase in risk for lower extremity PAD with earlier onset and faster progression.[20] PAD in patients with diabetes also typically affects the macro- and microvasculature of both lower extremities. Patients with diabetes diagnosis of greater than 10 years duration are at increased risk for lower extremity complications such as peripheral neuropathy, diabetic foot infection, and Charcot neuropathy.[21,22] Presence and history of all of these conditions should be inquired in a patient with diabetes.

Physical Examination

Physical examination of the lower extremity begins with visual assessment and pulse palpation. Findings on visual assessment that can heighten suspicion of a diagnosis of PAD include tar staining of the fingernails from smoking; surgical scars consistent with previous vascular procedures/surgeries on the neck, chest, abdomen, and lower extremities; and scars from previous healed wounds and amputated limbs or digits. The presence of active wounds should also be noted, particularly in areas of bony prominence and in between and on the distal aspects of the toes. Another test to perform is the Buerger's test. This is done by elevating the extremity approximately 45 to 60° from a supine position for 2 minutes and then in a dependent position for 2 minutes. Pallor on elevation and reactive hyperemia, also known as dependent rubor, is a positive Buerger sign, indicating distal or multisegmental arterial disease.[1,4,19,23] Although commonly performed, assessing lower extremity temperature and capillary refill time are not reliable indicators for PAD.[1] The presence of peripheral neuropathy should also be assessed, particularly in patients with diabetes, as its presence can mask symptoms of intermittent claudication and rest pain.[11,21]

Palpation and auscultation of the femoral, popliteal, posterior tibial, and dorsalispedis arteries should then be performed and is recommended in the guidelines by the International Working Group on the Diabetic Foot and the American Diabetes Association.[1,4,18,19] The popliteal pulse is relatively difficult to palpate. If it is easily felt this may indicate a popliteal aneurysm, which should be confirmed with an ultrasound study.[1] Lower extremity pulse palpation can be graded as follows: 0, absent; 1, diminished; 2, normal; or 4, bounding or simply as present or absent.[4] Although pulse palpation is not a sensitive tool for detection of PAD, absence of a palpable pulse has an excellent specificity for detection of PAD.[11] A significant difference in the amount of palpable pulses was found between patients with a normal ABI (mean 3.4), those with an ABI greater than or equal to 1.4 (mean 2.24) and those with an ABI less than or equal to 0.9 (mean 1.74). One or more missing or weak pedal pulses was found to have a significantly more sensitive and better negative predictive value than ABI less than 0.9 in predicting the presence of PAD.[19] Auscultation of a femoral bruit and absence of pedal pulses were both found to predict the presence of PAD.[9,15,18,19,24] Presence of a femoral bruit was found to be a risk factor for PAD independent of the presence of other cardiovascular risk factors.[15] Presence of all 4 pedal pulses was determined to be negative for PAD (sensitivity 72%, specificity 72%, positive predictive value 26%, negative predictive value 95%).[5] Combined with lack of a femoral bruit, the specificity increases to 98% for the absence of PAD.[9]

Pulse palpation is not without its faults though. For patients with more than or equal to 3 palpable pedal pulses, only 26% had PAD. Patients with diabetes and hypertension and active tobacco users were more likely to have a true positive or false negative for the presence of PAD.[5] Pulses can also be palpable in patients with PAD and affected by room temperature and the skill level of the provider performing the examination in addition to being nonpalpable due to congenital absence of the artery.[5,13,19,25–27] Complaints of intermittent claudication and pulse examination and auscultation taken individually have a low sensitivity and high specificity for detecting PAD (**Table 1**). Combination of these history and physical examination findings

Table 1
Detection of ankle-brachial index less than or equal to 0.9 based on intermittent claudication and pulse examination

Presence of History and Pulse Examination Finding	Sensitivity (%)	Specificity (%)	PPV (%)	NPV (%)	Accuracy (%)
Claudication	79	68	35	92	69
Palpable DP only	64	81	43	91	78
Palpable PT only	70	83	49	92	81
Palpable DP and PT	73	92	66	94	88
Femoral bruit only	36	92	51	86	82
Palpable DP and PT and no femoral bruit	58	98	81	95	94

Abbreviations: DP, dorsalis pedis; NPV, negative predictive value; PPV, positive predictive value; PT, posterior tibial.

Adapted from Armstrong DW, Tobin C, Matangi MF. The accuracy of the physical examination for the detection of lower extremity peripheral arterial disease. Can J Cardiol. 2010;26(10):e346–e350; with permission.

improve the accuracy of PAD detection, warranting the necessity of a thorough history and physical examination if the presence of PAD is a concern.[9]

Concerning findings on lower extremity pulse palpation examination warrants further evaluation through the use of a handheld Doppler. An 8-MHz handheld Doppler can be used to assess the posterior tibial and dorsalis pedis arteries as well as their connection at the pedal arch within the first intermetatarsal space of the foot. The probe should be held at an approximately 60° angle to the skin pointing in the direction of blood flow. It can then be manipulated to hear the clearest sound. The probe should be held so it is just in contact with the skin; holding the probe with excessive pressure to the skin can obliterate the arterial signal.[1] The arterial signal heard with a handheld Doppler is classified as triphasic, biphasic, or monophasic.[1] A triphasic signal is the audible signal heard from the 3 components of a normal waveform: high forward flow during systole due to left ventricular contraction, transient reversal of flow in early diastole due to reflection from a high-resistance outflow bed, and forward flow resulting from reflection from a closed aortic valve during late diastole. Biphasic waveforms result from loss of the audible signal of transient reversal of flow. A monophasic signal refers to forward flow only.[28] Audible handheld Doppler has a reported sensitivity of 42.8%, specificity of 97.5%, negative predictive value of 94.10%, and positive predictive value of 65.2% in predicting the presence of significant PAD.[29]

Lack of, or inadequate, training, inexperience, and time constraints account for the primary limitation of handheld Doppler use and correct interpretation of the audible signal heard.[12,30] Although studies conflict on the ability of clinicians of various years of experience to correctly interpret the audible signal heard, monophasic signal was the one most often correctly identified and the signal most concerning for PAD.[28,30] Other limitations of handheld Doppler use in assessing arterial signals are patient factors such as the presence of excessive edema, adipose tissue, fibrosis, and anatomic variations in artery location.[12] This can also cause difficulties in obtaining an ABI as discussed later.

Routine Noninvasive Vascular Studies

Ankle pressure and the ankle brachial index

Any abnormal findings on history and physical examination should be evaluated further with diagnostic testing to confirm the diagnosis of PAD. Obtaining an ABI is typically the initial test recommended in clinical guidelines.[4,5,8,14,18] The ABI is a measure of the systolic blood pressure of the posterior tibial or dorsalis pedis artery divided by the systolic blood pressure of the brachial artery. A resting ABI is typically first performed in which the patient is in a supine position and upper and lower extremity systolic blood pressure measurements are taken after a period of rest.[13] The systolic blood pressure of the upper and lower extremities should be equivalent with an ABI of 1.0 when PAD is not present.[20] An ABI less than or equal to 0.9 has a 90% sensitivity and 98% specificity for detection of stenosis of greater than or equal to 50% in the proximal lower limb, consistent with a diagnosis of PAD.[7,9] Variations in the number obtained aid in diagnosis and determination of severity of PAD (**Table 2**). The test is quick and easy to perform and involves minimal direct risk to the patient.[17] Controversy exists in using the ABI to screen asymptomatic patients due to the lack of evidence in the literature that support the benefit of reduced morbidity and mortality.[31] Although the direct risk of an ABI is minimal, indirect risks can include complications associated with administration of medications to treat hypertension and hyperlipidemia, exposure to contrast reagents if more invasive vascular studies ordered, and the potential anxiety created for the patient due to a false-positive reading.[17]

The main limitation of the ABI test is that it only provides information at the level of the artery being assessed and can be inaccurate due to systemic conditions affecting sensation, collateralization, and rigidity and presence of the vessel as well as recent tobacco use and caffeine intake.[1-3,13,16,20,31-34] A meta-analysis of 20 studies (2376 patients) found ABI to have a low prognostic accuracy in predicting lower extremity wounds that would heal (sensitivity 48%, specificity 52%). The ability to predict whether lower extremity amputation would occur was only slightly better (sensitivity 52%, specificity 73%).[31] ABI sensitivity in diagnosing PAD also varies in patients with diabetes and peripheral vascular disease versus those with diabetes and no peripheral vascular disease (100% vs 35% to 73%). ABI sensitivity and specificity are lower due to calcium build up within the lower extremity arteries, which makes the vessel noncompressible resulting in a falsely elevated ankle pressures.[2,3,20,31,33] This can occur in patients of older age, men, those with end-stage renal disease and rheumatoid arthritis, and tobacco users, although this is most often the concern in patients with diabetes.[2,9,19,32,35] Hardening of the arteries can result in an ABI result greater than or equal to 0.9 and palpable pedal pulses in the face of PAD. This is

Table 2	
Diagnosis of peripheral arterial disease and severity based on ankle-brachial index results	
Presence of PAD and Severity	**ABI Result**
Normal	1.0–1.3
PAD diagnosis	≤0.9
Falsely elevated	>1.3
Mild to moderate PAD	0.4–0.9
Severe PAD	<0.4

Data from Khan TH, Farooqui FA, Niazi K. Critical review of the ankle brachial index. Curr Cardiol Rev. 2008;4(2):101–106.

particularly problematic in patients with active lower extremity ulcerations in which un-diagnosed and untreated PAD can lead to delayed healing and increased risk of amputation.[19] More than 50% of patients with diabetes and peripheral neuropathy with an ABI between 0.9 and 1.3 have PAD. The prevalence of PAD increases to 85% when the ABI is greater than or equal to 1.4.[20] Additional vascular studies are rec-ommended in these circumstances.[19]

In patients with heel ulcerations, more than 50% of the ABI results obtained were based on the dorsalis pedis artery, which is not the primary vascular supply of the angiosome of the heel.[36] In addition, the methods in which the ABI is obtained and calculated can produce different results.[1,3,5,11,15,16,37] An oscillometric ABI has been reported to have a higher sensitivity and specificity compared with a manual Doppler ABI (97% and 98%, respectively, vs 95% and 56%).[3] The traditional method of calcu-lating an ABI involves dividing the higher brachial systolic pressure by the higher of the posterior tibial or dorsalis pedis arteries.[1,7,11,15,16] However, various methods do exist.[5,7,32,37,38] Dividing the lower of the posterior tibial or dorsalis pedis systolic pres-sures by the higher brachial artery may identify more patients at risk for all-cause and cardiovascular mortality.[7,32,37,38] Performing an ABI after exercises may also assist in PAD diagnosis if there are concerns regarding the accuracy of the resting ABI result. The ABI result following exercise will decrease in respect to the patient's resting ABI if PAD is present. Patients can do a formal treadmill test for exercise or mimic a treadmill test by performing 20 heel-toe raises.[1]

Toe pressure and the toe brachial index
When the ABI is considered to be falsely elevated, toe pressures and calculation of the toe brachial index are often used, as the digital arteries are less likely to be affected by medial calcinosis.[2,13,20,39,40] Systolic toe pressure has been reported to have 100% sensitivity in detecting PAD whereas systolic ankle pressure is just greater than 50%.[20] Using a cut-off of 30 mmHg, systolic toe pressure measurements have a sensitivity and specificity of 15% and 97%, respectively,predicting adequate perfu-sion available for healing (positive predictive value 67% and negative predictive value 77%).[31] A toe brachial index (TBI) can also be obtained in which the systolic pressure of the toe is divided by the systolic pressure of the brachial artery. A review of 22 studies reported that a TBI between 0.54 and 0.75 indicates PAD with a sensitivity of 90% to 100% and specificity between 65% and 100%.[3] A TBI less than 0.7 has been reported in association with intermittent claudication and less than 0.2 in asso-ciation with rest pain.[3]

Limitations of toe pressure and TBI are similar to those of the ABI; results only pro-vide information of pressure measurement at the level of the digit and can be inaccu-rate due to size of the cuff used for testing, rigidity of the vessel, room and skin temperature, and patient factors such as female gender, tobacco and caffeine use, lack of designation of a consistent cut-off denoting the presence of PAD and lack of high-quality and contradictory literature to support its use as a screening or diagnostic test for PAD.[19,39,41] Use of a narrower cuff has been reported to result in higher toe pressure readings, whereas female gender is associated with lower toe pressure read-ings.[41] A systematic review and meta-analysis of 8 studies (909 patients) in the utility of toe pressure to predict healing of diabetic foot ulcerations reported a pooled sensi-tivity and specificity of 86% and 56%, respectively, using a cut-off value of 30 mm Hg.[40] A systematic review of 7 studies (566 lower limbs) reported the pooled sensitivity and specificity of TBI to detect PAD to range from 45% to 100% and 16% to 100%, respectively.[40] Heterogeneity existed between the studies, including variation in the cut-off TBI value used to signify PAD. TBI values consistent with PAD currently range from less than 0.54 to 0.75.[41] Approximately 25% of patients with a toe pressure less than 30 mmHg have been reported to heal lower extremity ulcerations, whereas the same percentage with a toe pressure greater than 91 mmHg has delayed healing.[41] In addition, although obtaining a TBI is recommended when ABI results are falsely elevated due to the theory that the digital arteries are less often affected, this was not confirmed in a study comparing ABI and TBI results obtained in patients with diabetes and those without diabetes. Digital artery calcification was evident on 24% to 40% of plain film radiographs of the feet of patients with diabetes despite plain film radiographs having a reported limited sensitivity in detecting arterial calcification.[2] Obtaining a toe pressure and TBI is also not possible when digital ulceration is present or the patient lacks digits due to previous amputation.[31,33,34,42]

Transcutaneous oxygen pressure measurement

Transcutaneous oxygen pressure measurement (TCOM) is one of the most common skin perfusion measurements performed. TCOM measures capillary oxygen tension via probes placed on the skin that are heated to approximately 43°C. This causes local vasodilation and oxygen diffusion to the skin surface for measurement. A meta-analysis of the ability of 8 vascular studies to predict adequate perfusion for healing of a diabetic foot ulceration found that TCOM results were better able to predict wounds that would heal and the necessity for amputation compared with results of an ABI.[31]

Limitations of TCOM use are the variation in cut-off points used to determine adequate perfusion for healing, patient factors that can affect results, time and skilled personnel required to perform the examination, and that vascular assessment is provided at the point of probe placement only with no clearly defined cut-off value that indicates adequate perfusion for healing.[33,42,43] TCOM cut-off values to signify adequate perfusion range from 25 mmHg to 50 mmHg.[24,44] A TCOM greater than 25 mmHg has a reported 92% specificity for predicting wound healing. A TCOM of greater than 30 mmHg has been reported to be highly accurate in predicting symptom management and wound healing after implementation of conservative or surgical measures. A TCOM of greater than 40 mmHg is recommended as a cut-off value to signify adequate perfusion for healing if severe gangrene or calcaneal tissue loss is present.[24] One study found that a dorsal TCOM greater than 30 mmHg in a patient with a heal ulcer had CLI when a corresponding rearfoot TCOM was performed. Mean rearfoot TCOM results in these patients with heel ulceration and dorsal TCOM greater than or equal to 30 mmHg had a rearfoot TCOM result of 21 mmHg.[44] The TransAtlantic Inter-Society Consensus designated a TCOM less than 50 mmHg as objective criteria for CLI.[44] Patient factors that can adversely affect TCOM results include edema, dry flaky skin, maceration, callused or plantar skin, cellulitis, and probe placement over bones and tendons.[24,44]

Skin perfusion pressure

Skin perfusion pressure (SPP) measurements are most often obtained by use of a laser Doppler sensor placed on the foot or toe, whereas a blood pressure sensor is placed at the ankle or toe, respectively. The pressure at which skin perfusion returns following vascular occlusion and controlled release is the SPP. Multiple sites can be tested, one at a time, taking about 10 to 15 minutes per site. The skin can also be warmed to 42°C if necessary.[45–47] SPP has been reported to not be effected by artery calcification.[47] The ability to perform an SPP was found to be universal in 211 patients (403 limbs), whereas only 351 (87%) limbs, 367 (91%) limbs, and 380 (94%) limbs could have ankle pressue, toe pressure, and TCOM performed, respectively.[34]

Limitations of the SPP include the ability to provide vascular assessment at the site of blood pressure cuff placement, skin and body temperature, sympathetic tone, limb position, time and skilled personnel required to perform the examination, and lack of a clearly defined cut-off value that indicates adequate perfusion for healing.[46,48–50] Having the patient seated with their lower extremities extended along the table without a bend in the knee has been reported to be the optimal position for obtaining SPP measurements. Performing an SPP with the patient seated and the legs in a dependent position has been shown to result in elevated SPP results.[49,50] Although an SPP greater than 30 mmHg has a reported 100% sensitivity and 97% specificity of determining healing potential following a major lower extremity amputation, this decreases when looking at the potential to heal lower extremity wounds and partial foot amputations (61%–85% sensitivity, 67%–80%, respectively).[45,46] Increasing the cut-off SPP value will decrease sensitivity and increase specificity. A meta-analysis comparing a cut-off SPP value of 30 mmHg and 40 mmHg reported a decrease in sensitivity (79.9%–67.1%) and increase in specificity (78.2%–84.2%) with a larger SPP cut-off value.[47] Thus, an SPP of 30 to 40 mmHg has been deemed to predict the presence of adequate perfusion for healing.[42,45–47,51–54] Further designation is listed in **Table 3**. A cut-off value of greater than 70 mmHg has also been recommended as the minimum, indicating adequate perfusion and minimization for the potential for amputation as well as reduction in mortality rates for patients with end-stage renal disease on hemodialysis.[54,55]

Novel Vascular Studies

Hyperspectral and near-infrared imaging

Hyperspectral imaging measures tissue oxygenation levels. Tissue oxygenation saturation has been used for decades to determine cerebral perfusion, skin perfusion in sepsis and septic shock, irritant-induced inflammation, ischemia-reperfusion injury, the effect of ultraviolet irradiation, optical detection of cancer, and diagnosis of PAD.[56,57] The signal received is based on the oxygen-carrying status of blood within the microcirculation.[31,58] A systematic review of these imaging modalities found them to be a valuable measure of PAD through objective assessment of tissue mismatch in oxygen demand and supply in the area imaged.[59] The amount of deoxygenated hemoglobin present, postocclusive resaturation rates, and recovery times have been found to be representative of microvascular function and best correlate with ABI results.[56,60] Angiosome mapping based on imaging results from these studies, as opposed to angiography-based angiosome assessment, was found to have a sensitivity and specificity of 88% and 69%, respectively, in predicting arterial ulceration location.[48,58] This is hypothesized to be due to collateralization and other factors altering microcirculatory flow in patients with PAD, resulting in alteration of the major arterial supply to an angiosome.[58]

Table 3
Diagnosis of peripheral arterial disease and severity and average time to wound healing based on skin pressure perfusion results

Presence of PAD and Severity	SPP Result (mmHg)	Average Time to Wound Healing (d)
Normal	>50	235
Mild to moderate PAD	31–50	98
Severe PAD	≤30	52

Use of hyperspectral imaging during initial evaluation and through serial assessment of wounds in patients with type I and type II diabetes has also been shown to better predict wound resolution compared with the gold standard of wound measurements and 50% reduction in wound size at 4 weeks. These findings suggest that hyperspectral imaging is better able to predict wound resolution earlier, enabling physicians to begin earlier aggressive treatment of expedited wound resolution if deemed necessary.[56,61,62] A healing index, a proprietary device-calculation measurement in one type of hyperspectral imaging system, is obtained based on readings obtained from the wound base and a 0.5 to 2.5 cm margin of the periwound skin. A healing index greater than 0 had a sensitivity and specificity of 93% and 86%, respectively, and a 90% to 93% positive predictive value and 86% negative predictive value for wound resolution.

Although hyperspectral imaging is obtained in a noncontact, noninvasive fashion, other near-infrared imaging modalities require intravenous access for injection of dyes that fluoresces under near-infrared light. Parameters for assessment of tissue perfusion are most often based on time and intensity of the fluoresce signal produced; techniques in which these parameters are obtained varied on the device utilized. Devices that function with a larger dose of fluorescent dye use a more binary measurement system based on time and intensity of fluorescence onset and regress, as these devices do not perform any analysis on the images obtained. Other systems use smaller doses of fluorescent dye and provide analytical parameters that allow for subtle assessment of fluorescence signal onset, filling pattern, and regression[26,57] (Table 4).

A systematic review of 23 articles on near-infrared imaging, the majority using indocyanine green for the fluorescent dye, found it to be a valuable tool in diagnosing PAD or CLI, visualizing regional perfusion changes following revascularization procedures, providing early prediction on wounds not likely to heal, and assessing accurate level of amputation most likely to heal.[57] The parameters of $T_{1/2}$, PDE_{10}, and Td 90% were reported to be the most beneficial in vascular assessment. Near-infrared imaging parameters have a reported sensitivity and specificity range of 67% to 100% and 72% to 100%, respectively, for diagnosing PAD or CLI. ABI results have been shown to have significant correlations with $T_{1/2}$, Td 90%, T_{max}, Td 75%, and intensity reading at 60 seconds, with Td 90% determined to be the most significant variable. A Td 90% of 25 seconds diagnostically predict PAD with a sensitivity and specificity of 82.6% and 73.3%, respectively.[63,64] $T_{1/2}$ has been able to distinguish between Fontaine II and IV[65] (Table 5). A PDE_{10} of 28 was found to be the optimal cut-off for detecting CLI defined as a TCOM less than or equal to 30 mmHg with a sensitivity and specificity of 100% and 86.6%, respectively.[66] All vascular assessment parameters have been noted to increase following successful vascular intervention, whereas no change occurred in patients in whom revascularization was not successful.[57] Lack of fluorescence in the wound bed and mottled appearance of signal has also been associated with delayed healing of wounds.[33] Review of the raw imaging sequence itself, particularly in systems using smaller doses of fluorescent dye, have also been reported to be of utility in diagnosing local ischemia and PAD. Patients with delayed time to onset of fluorescence and a mottled pattern of fluorescence filling have been noted to be characteristic of PAD.[26,67]

Benefits of this type of imaging is that it is easy; rapid to perform; provides real-time, site-specific vascular assessment; has reproducible results; is not affected by factors that limit results of routine noninvasive vascular studies; and allows for repeated study/image analysis without the need for repeated studies in addition to some modalities offering noncontact and noninvasive image capture.[26,33,42,48,56–58,67–71]

Table 4
Near-infrared imaging vascular assessment parameters

Parameter	Definition	Self-Determined Parameter	Device-Determined Parameter
Ingress	Magnitude of increase in fluorescence from baseline to max intensity		X
Ingress rate	Rate of fluorescence intensity increase from baseline to max intensity		X
Egress	Magnitude of decrease in fluorescence from max intensity to end of fluorescence		X
Egress rate	Rate of fluorescence intensity decrease from max intensity to end of fluorescence		X
T_{max}	Time from onset to maximum fluorescence intensity	X	
PDE_{10}	Intensity of fluorescence 10 s after onset of fluorescence	X	
$T_{1/2}$	Time to half maximum intensity	X	
Td90%	Time elapsed from maximum fluorescence intensity to 90% intensity	X	
Td75%	Time elapsed from maximum fluorescence intensity to 75% intensity	X	

Adapted from van den Hoven P, Ooms S, van Manen L, et al. A systematic review of the use of near-infrared fluorescence imaging in patients with peripheral artery disease. J Vasc Surg. 2019 Jul;70(1):286-297.e1; with permission.

Limitations primarily exist in regard to factors that can lead to altered fluorescence signal reading such as positioning during image capture, room lighting, presence of infection, inflammation, thickened skin, increased melanin content, angiogenesis, tissue within the wound base, such as eschar, slough, coagulum, and advanced tissue products, and variations in depth of penetration of the imaging device.[26,48,57,61,66,67] The positive predictive value of these imaging modalities was found to decrease by 6% in the presence of underlying osteomyelitis.[61] Algorithms are continuing to be

Table 5
Fontaine classification system[65]

Stage	Symptoms
I	Asymptomatic, incomplete blood vessel obstruction
II	Mild claudication pain in limb
IIA	Claudication at a distance >200 m
IIB	Claudication at a distance <200 m
III	Rest pain, mostly in the feet
IV	Necrosis and/or gangrene of the limb

created to offset difference in readings due to melanin content in the skin. These factors, in addition to limited comparison studies, may be the reason for lack of correlation of hyperspectral and near-infrared imaging study results with routine noninvasive vascular studies.[71] Other limitations involve those devices that require intravenous access for imaging, expense of the device, and time and staff training required for proper imaging capture and analysis.

SUMMARY

Current guidelines vary on whether or not asymptomatic patients should be screened for PAD.[4,8,14,18,39] In treating patients with a lower extremity wound, the primary concern shifts from the risk of PAD progression and mortality related to cardiovascular events to wound healing to prevent limb loss, an independent risk factor for increased morbidity and mortality. Vascular assessment of these patients typically relies on standard history and physical examination findings, which could delay appropriate intervention. Studies have shown that history and physical examination findings are insufficient to diagnosis PAD and recommend further vascular testing to aid in the diagnosis.[3–5,9–13,17,19,20,39,40] However, which tests to obtain remains controversial, given the limitations of routine noninvasive vascular studies.[27] The need for quantitative and accurate information of adequate blood supply is critical for timely intervention if necessary.[69]

Although limited studies have looked at the sensitivity and specificity of combining history and physical examination findings with vascular study results in accurately diagnosing PAD, recommendation has been made to combine various vascular study results to improve accuracy. Some studies recommend use of toe pressure/TBI and SPP over ABI and TCOM when possible.[27,42,70] An SPP greater than or equal to 40 mmHg in conjunction with a toe pressure greater than or equal to 30 mmHg was found to accurately predict the ability to heal lower extremity wounds in patients with PAD.[34,42,47] Other studies recommend combination of physical examination findings, with TCOM less than 40 mmHg or with SPP and TCOM results.[43,47] Novel vascular assessment modalities seem to supplement clinical assessment and routine noninvasive vascular studies, given that results are site specific and not limited by factors that can make results of noninvasive vascular studies unreliable.[69] The result of this review suggests that a thorough history focused on specific risk factors, pulse palpation, auscultation, and Doppler evaluation combined with hemodynamic measurements may help provide a more accurate diagnosis of PAD. Novel vascular assessment modalities may be an option to consider in patients in whom the accuracy of routine noninvasive vascular study results is questioned.

ACKNOWLEDGMENTS

The author wishes to thank Valerie Marmolejo, DPM, MS, Medical Writer, from Scriptum Medica (www.scriptummedica.com) for her assistance in preparation of this article.

DISCLOSURE

The author has nothing to disclose.

REFERENCES

1. Bailey MA, Griffin KJ, Scott DJ. Clinical assessment of patients with peripheral arterial disease. SeminInterventRadiol 2014;31(4):292–9.

2. Stoekenbroek RM, Ubbink DT, Reekers JA, et al. Hide and seek: does the toe-brachial index allow for earlier recognition of peripheral arterial disease in diabetic patients? Eur J VascEndovasc Surg 2015;49(2):192–8.

3. ShabaniVaraki E, Gargiulo GD, Penkala S, et al. Peripheral vascular disease assessment in the lower limb: a review of current and emerging non-invasive diagnostic methods. Biomed EngOnline 2018;17(1):61.

4. Writing Committee Members, Gerhard-Herman MD, Gornik HL, et al. 2016 AHA/ACC guideline on the management of patients with lower extremity peripheral artery disease: executive summary. Vasc Med 2017;22(3):NP1–43.

5. Londero LS, Lindholt JS, Thomsen MD, et al. Pulse palpation is an effective method for population-based screening to exclude peripheral arterial disease. J Vasc Surg 2016;63(5):1305–10.

6. Robbins JM, Strauss G, Aron D, et al. Mortality rates and diabetic foot ulcers: is it time to communicate mortality risk to patients with diabetic foot ulceration? J Am Podiatr Med Assoc 2008;98(6):489–93.

7. Khan TH, Farooqui FA, Niazi K. Critical review of the ankle brachial index. Curr-Cardiol Rev 2008;4(2):101–6.

8. Guirguis-Blake JM, Evans CV, Redmond N, et al. Screening for peripheral artery disease using the ankle-brachial index: updated evidence report and systematic review for the US preventive services task force. JAMA 2018;320(2):184–96.

9. Armstrong DW, Tobin C, Matangi MF. The accuracy of the physical examination for the detection of lower extremity peripheral arterial disease. Can J Cardiol 2010;26(10):e346–50.

10. Tickner A, Klinghard C, Arnold JF, et al. Total contact cast use in patients with peripheral arterial disease: a case series and systematic review. Wounds 2018; 30(2):49–56.

11. Collins TC, Suarez-Almazor M, Peterson NJ. An absent pulse is not sensitive for the early detection of peripheral arterial disease. Fam Med 2006;38(1):38–42.

12. Tehan PE, Chuter VH. Use of hand-held Doppler ultrasound examination by podiatrists: a reliability study. J FootAnkle Res 2015;8:36.

13. Bonham P. Measuring toe pressures using a portable photoplethysmograph to detect arterial disease in high-risk patients: an overview of the literature. Ostomy Wound Manage 2011;57(11):36–44.

14. Hingorani A, LaMuraglia GM, Henke P, et al. The management of diabetic foot: A clinical practice guideline by the Society for Vascular Surgery in collaboration with the American Podiatric Medical Association and the Society for Vascular Medicine. J Vasc Surg 2016;63(2 Suppl):3S–21S.

15. Cournot M, Boccalon H, Cambou JP, et al. Accuracy of the screening physical examination to identify subclinical atherosclerosis and peripheral arterial disease in asymptomatic subjects. J Vasc Surg 2007;46(6):1215–21.

16. Casey S, Lanting S, Oldmeadow C, et al. The reliability of the ankle brachial index: a systematic review. J FootAnkle Res 2019;12:39.

17. Alahdab F, Wang AT, Elraiyah TA, et al. A systematic review for the screening for peripheral arterial disease in asymptomatic patients. J Vasc Surg 2015;61(3 Suppl):42S–53S.

18. American Diabetes Association. Peripheral arterial disease in people with diabetes. Diabetes Care 2003;26(12):3333–41.

19. Schaper NC, Andros G, Apelqvist J, et al. Diagnosis and treatment of peripheral arterial disease in diabetic patients with a foot ulcer. A progress report of the International Working Group on the Diabetic Foot. DiabetesMetab Res Rev 2012; 28(Suppl 1):218–24.

20. Aubert CE, Cluzel P, Kemel S, et al. Influence of peripheral vascular calcification on efficiency of screening tests for peripheral arterial occlusive disease in diabetes—a cross-sectional study. Diabet Med 2014;31(2):192–9.
21. Abouhamda A, Alturkstani M, Jan Y. Lower sensitivity of ankle-brachial index measurements among people suffering with diabetes-associated vascular disorders: A systematic review. SAGEOpen Med 2019;7. 2050312119835038.
22. Marmolejo VS, Arnold JF, Ponticello M, et al. Charcot foot: clinical clues, diagnostic strategies, and treatment principles. Am FamPhysician 2018;97(9):594–9.
23. Insall RL, Davies RJ, Prout WG. Significance of Buerger's test in the assessment of lower limb ischaemia. J R Soc Med 1989;82(12):729–31.
24. Ballard JL, Eke CC, Bunt TJ, et al. A prospective evaluation of transcutaneous oxygen measurements in the management of diabetic foot problems. J Vasc Surg 1995;22(4):485–90 [discussion: 490–2].
25. Álvaro-Afonso FJ, García-Morales E, Molines-Barroso RJ, et al. Interobserver reliability of the ankle-brachial index, toe-brachial index and distal pulse palpation in patients with diabetes. DiabVasc Dis Res 2018;15(4):344–7.
26. Marmolejo VS, Arnold JF. The ability of fluorescence angiography to detect local ischemia in patients with heel ulceration. FootAnkle Spec 2018;11(3):269–76.
27. Barshes NR, Flores E, Belkin M, et al. The accuracy and cost-effectiveness of strategies used to identify peripheral artery disease among patients with diabetic foot ulcers. J Vasc Surg 2016;64(6):1682–90.e3.
28. Omarjee L, Stivalet O, Hoffmann C, et al. Heterogeneity of Doppler waveform description is decreased with the use of a dedicated classification. Vasa 2018; 47(6):471–4.
29. Alavi A, Sibbald RG, Nabavizadeh R, et al. Audible handheld Doppler ultrasound determines reliable and inexpensive exclusion of significant peripheral arterial disease. Vascular 2015;23(6):622–9.
30. Young M, Birch I, Potter CA, et al. A comparison of the Doppler ultrasound interpretation by student and registered podiatrists. J FootAnkle Res 2013;6(1):25.
31. Wang Z, Hasan R, Firwana B, et al. A systematic review and meta-analysis of tests to predict wound healing in diabetic foot. J Vasc Surg 2016;63(2 Suppl): 29S–36S.e1-2.
32. Bunte MC, Jacob J, Nudelman B, et al. Validation of the relationship between ankle-brachial and toe-brachial indices and infragenicular arterial patency in critical limb ischemia. Vasc Med 2015;20(1):23–9.
33. Arnold JF. Is there adequate perfusion for healing? what routine noninvasive vascular studies are missing? Wounds 2018;30(9):E89–92.
34. Tsai FW, Tulsyan N, Jones DN, et al. Skin perfusion pressure of the foot is a good substitute for toe pressure in the assessment of limb ischemia. J Vasc Surg 2000; 32(1):32–6.
35. Nam SC, Han SH, Lim SH, et al. Factors affecting the validity of ankle-brachial index in the diagnosis of peripheral arterial obstructive disease. Angiology 2010;61(4):392–6.
36. Crowell A, Meyr AJ. Accuracy of the ankle-brachial index in the assessment of arterial perfusion of heel pressure injuries. Wounds 2017;29(2):51–5.
37. Nead KT, Cooke JP, Olin JW, et al. Alternative ankle-brachial index method identifies additional at-risk individuals. J Am CollCardiol 2013;62(6):553–9.
38. Jeevanantham V, Chehab B, Austria E, et al. Comparison of accuracy of two different methods to determine ankle-brachial index to predict peripheral arterial disease severity confirmed by angiography. Am J Cardiol 2014;114(7):1105–10.

39. Society for Vascular Surgery Lower Extremity Guidelines Writing Group, Conte MS, Pomposelli FB, et al. Society for Vascular Surgery practice guidelines for atherosclerotic occlusive disease of the lower extremities: management of asymptomatic disease and claudication [published correction appears in J Vasc Surg. 2015 May;61(5):1382]. J Vasc Surg 2015;61(3 Suppl):2S–41S.
40. Tehan PE, Santos D, Chuter VH. A systematic review of the sensitivity and specificity of the toe-brachial index for detecting peripheral artery disease. Vasc Med 2016;21(4):382–9.
41. Trevethan R. Toe systolic pressures and toe-brachial indices: uses, abuses, and shades of gray. Blood Press Monit 2019;24(2):45–51.
42. Yamada T, Ohta T, Ishibashi H, et al. Clinical reliability and utility of skin perfusion pressure measurement in ischemic limbs–comparison with other noninvasive diagnostic methods. J Vasc Surg 2008;47(2):318–23.
43. Arsenault KA, Al-Otaibi A, Devereaux PJ, et al. The use of transcutaneous oximetry to predict healing complications of lower limb amputations: a systematic review and meta-analysis. Eur J VascEndovasc Surg 2012;43(3):329–36.
44. Izzo V, Meloni M, Fabiano S, et al. Rearfoot transcutaneous oximetry is a useful tool to highlight ischemia of the heel. CardiovascInterventRadiol 2017;40(1): 120–4.
45. Adera HM, James K, Castronuovo JJ Jr, et al. Prediction of amputation wound healing with skin perfusion pressure. J Vasc Surg 1995;21(5):823–8 [discussion: 828–9].
46. Castronuovo JJ Jr, Adera HM, Smiell JM, et al. Skin perfusion pressure measurement is valuable In the diagnosis of critical limb ischemia. J Vasc Surg 1997; 26(4):629–37.
47. Pan X, You C, Chen G, et al. Skin perfusion pressure for the prediction of wound healing in critical limb ischemia: a meta-analysis. Arch Med Sci 2018;14(3): 481–7.
48. Boezeman RP, Becx BP, van den Heuvel DA, et al. Monitoring of foot oxygenation with near-infrared spectroscopy in patients with critical limb ischemia undergoing percutaneous transluminal angioplasty: a pilot study. Eur J VascEndovasc Surg 2016;52(5):650–6.
49. Shinozaki N. Effect of body position on skin perfusion pressure in patients with severe peripheral arterial disease. Circ J 2012;76(12):2863–6.
50. Kawasaki T, Uemura T, Matsuo K, et al. The effect of different positions on lower limbs skin perfusion pressure. Indian J Plast Surg 2013;46(3):508–12.
51. Urabe G, Yamamoto K, Onozuka A, et al. Skin perfusion pressure is a useful tool for evaluating outcome of ischemic foot ulcers with conservative therapy. Ann Vasc Dis 2009;2(1):21–6.
52. Watanabe Y, Onozuka A, Obitsu Y, et al. Skin perfusion pressure measurement to assess improvement in peripheral circulation after arterial reconstruction for critical limb ischemia. Ann Vasc Dis 2011;4(3):235–40.
53. Tsuji Y, Hiroto T, Kitano I, et al. Importance of skin perfusion pressure in treatment of critical limb ischemia. Wounds 2008;20(4):95–100.
54. Suzuki K, Birnbaum Z, Lockhart R. Skin perfusion pressure and wound closure time in lower extremity wounds. J Am CollClinWound Spec 2018;9(1–3):14–8.
55. Hatakeyama S, Saito M, Ishigaki K, et al. Skin perfusion pressure is a prognostic factor in hemodialysis patients. Int J Nephrol 2012;2012:385274.
56. Khaodhiar L, Dinh T, Schomacker KT, et al. The use of medical hyperspectral technology to evaluate microcirculatory changes in diabetic foot ulcers and predict clinical outcomes. Diabetes Care 2007;30:903–10.

57. van den Hoven P, Ooms S, van Manen L, et al. A systematic review of the use of near-infrared fluorescence imaging in patients with peripheral artery disease. J Vasc Surg 2019;70(1):286–97.e1.

58. Kagaya Y, Ohura N, Suga H, et al. Real angiosome' assessment from peripheral tissue perfusion using tissue oxygen saturation foot-mapping in patients with critical limb ischemia. Eur J VascEndovasc Surg 2014;47(4):433–41.

59. Vardi M, Nini A. Near-infrared spectroscopy for evaluation of peripheral vascular disease. A systematic review of literature. Eur J VascEndovasc Surg 2008;35(1):68–74.

60. Chin JA, Wang EC, Kibbe MR. Evaluation of hyperspectral technology for assessing the presence and severity of peripheral artery disease. J Vasc Surg 2011;54(6):1679–88.

61. Nouvong A, Hoogwerf B, Mohler E, et al. Evaluation of diabetic foot ulcer healing with hyperspectral imaging of oxyhemoglobin and deoxyhemoglobin. Diabetes Care 2009;32(11):2056–61.

62. Neidrauer M, Zubkov L, Weingarten MS, et al. Near infrared wound monitor helps clinical assessment of diabetic foot ulcers. J DiabetesSci Technol 2010;4(4):792–8.

63. Igari K, Kudo T, Uchiyama H, et al. Indocyanine green angiography for the diagnosis of peripheral arterial disease with isolated infrapopliteal lesions. Ann Vasc Surg 2014;28(6):1479–84.

64. Igari K, Kudo T, Uchiyama H, et al. Intraarterial injection of indocyanine green for evaluation of peripheral blood circulation in patients with peripheral arterial disease. Ann Vasc Surg 2014;28(5):1280–5.

65. Hardman RL, Jazaeri O, Yi J, et al. Overview of classification systems in peripheral artery disease. SeminInterventRadiol 2014;31(4):378–88.

66. Terasaki H, Inoue Y, Sugano N, et al. A quantitative method for evaluating local perfusion using indocyanine green fluorescence imaging. Ann Vasc Surg 2013;27(8):1154–61.

67. Arnold JF, Roscum M. The EXPLORE trial: a feasibility study using fluorescence angiography to evaluate perfusion in the oxygen-rich environment. SurgTechnol Int 2016;29:61–79.

68. Goodall RJ, Langridge B, Onida S, et al. Current status of noninvasive perfusion assessment in individuals with diabetic foot ulceration. J Vasc Surg 2019;69(2):315–7.

69. Mukherjee R, Tewary S, Routray A. Diagnostic and prognostic utility of noninvasive multimodal imaging in chronic wound monitoring: a systematic review. J Med Syst 2017;41(3):46.

70. Lo T, Sample R, Moore P, et al. Prediction of wound healing outcome using skin perfusion pressure and transcutaneous oximetry: A single-center experience in 100 patients. Wounds 2009;21(11):310–6.

71. Jeffcoate WJ, Clark DJ, Savic N, et al. Use of HSI to measure oxygen saturation in the lower limb and its correlation with healing of foot ulcers in diabetes. Diabet Med 2015;32(6):798–802.

Moving?

Make sure your subscription moves with you!

To notify us of your new address, find your **Clinics Account Number** (located on your mailing label above your name), and contact customer service at:

Email: journalscustomerservice-usa@elsevier.com

800-654-2452 (subscribers in the U.S. & Canada)
314-447-8871 (subscribers outside of the U.S. & Canada)

Fax number: 314-447-8029

Elsevier Health Sciences Division
Subscription Customer Service
3251 Riverport Lane
Maryland Heights, MO 63043

*To ensure uninterrupted delivery of your subscription, please notify us at least 4 weeks in advance of move.

Printed and bound by CPI Group (UK) Ltd, Croydon, CR0 4YY

03/10/2024

01040401-0015